How to Perform Isometric Exercise for Seniors

Safe, Low-Impact Strength Training for Older Adults

Manuel Hayes

Table of Contents

Introduction

Have you ever watched younger people effortlessly maintaining their strength and flexibility, wishing you could do the same without the strain on your joints or the need for expensive gym equipment? Do you find yourself wanting to improve your balance, muscle tone, and overall fitness, but feel discouraged by high-impact workouts that seem unsuitable for your age? I completely understand those concerns.

Like many seniors, I used to believe that effective strength training was beyond my reach. Every time I considered starting a fitness routine, I'd hesitate, worried about injury or overwhelmed by complex exercise programs. But then I discovered the transformative power of isometric exercise, and it changed everything.

Imagine being able to significantly improve your strength, balance, and flexibility from the comfort of your own home, without any special equipment. Picture yourself confidently performing exercises that enhance your daily life, reduce the risk of falls, and keep you feeling young and vibrant. With "How to Perform Isometric Exercise for Seniors," you'll gain the knowledge and techniques to do just that.

This comprehensive guide is designed to empower you with safe, effective isometric exercises tailored specifically for older adults. Whether you're a complete beginner to fitness or looking to adapt your routine as you age, this book will take you from hesitant to confident in your ability to improve your health through exercise.

Here's what you'll discover within these pages:

- The science behind isometric exercise and why it's ideal for seniors
- How to assess your current fitness level and set achievable goals
- A wide range of isometric exercises for every part of your body
- Techniques for incorporating isometric training into your daily routine
- Strategies for progressing safely and avoiding common pitfalls
- Nutrition and recovery tips to support your new active lifestyle

By investing in this guide, you're not just buying a book – you're unlocking the potential to transform your health, maintain your independence, and enjoy a higher quality of life. You'll save money on gym memberships and personal trainers while gaining the satisfaction of taking control of your fitness journey.

So why let age hold you back when you can become the master of your own strength and flexibility? Dive in now, and discover how to improve your health, impress your doctor with your progress, and perhaps even inspire your peers to join you in this safe and effective form of exercise.

Are you ready to embrace the power of isometric exercise and start feeling stronger, more balanced, and more confident in your daily life? Let's embark on this exciting journey together and unlock the secrets of senior fitness through isometric training!

Chapter 1
Introduction to Isometric Exercise for Seniors

What Are Isometric Exercises?

Imagine holding a heavy book against a wall, your muscles working hard but not moving. That's the essence of isometric exercise - a form of strength training where you contract your muscles without changing their length or moving your joints. It's like pressing an immovable object or resisting an unstoppable force.

Why it's ideal for seniors:
- Low impact on joints
- Can be performed anywhere, anytime
- Requires no special equipment
- Highly effective for maintaining and building strength

Let's dive deeper into the science and benefits of isometric exercise:

The Science Behind Isometrics:
When you perform an isometric exercise, your muscles generate tension without shortening or lengthening. This static contraction:

1. Increases muscle fiber recruitment
2. Improves neuromuscular efficiency
3. Enhances muscle endurance
4. Strengthens tendons and ligaments

Imagine your muscles as a team of workers. In isometric exercise, you're asking every worker to show up and contribute, even though the overall "shape" of the team doesn't change.

Key Components of Isometric Exercise:

1. Duration: Typically held for 6-10 seconds
2. Intensity: Can be adjusted based on how hard you push or pull
3. Repetitions: Usually performed in sets of 5-10 holds
4. Rest periods: Crucial for recovery between sets

Troubleshooting Tip: If you experience muscle shaking during holds, reduce the intensity or duration. Gradual progression is key to building strength safely.

Types of Isometric Exercises:

1. Yielding Isometrics: Holding a weight or position against gravity
 Example: Wall sit or plank hold

2. Overcoming Isometrics: Pushing or pulling against an immovable object
 Example: Pushing against a wall or doorframe

3. Functional Isometrics: Holding a position in everyday movements
 Example: Pausing at the bottom of a sit-to-stand motion

Troubleshooting Tip: If you find one type of isometric exercise uncomfortable, try another. The key is finding exercises that challenge you without causing pain.

Benefits for Seniors:

1. Improved Muscle Strength: Particularly beneficial for maintaining strength in aging muscles

2. Enhanced Balance and Stability: Strengthens core and stabilizing muscles, reducing fall risk

3. Joint Health: Strengthens muscles around joints without stressing the joints themselves

4. Cardiovascular Health: Can lead to temporary increases in blood pressure, potentially improving overall cardiovascular function when done safely

5. Bone Density: May help maintain bone density, crucial for preventing osteoporosis

6. Accessibility: Can be performed by those with limited mobility or in small spaces

Troubleshooting Tip: If you have high blood pressure, consult your doctor before starting isometric exercises. They may recommend monitoring your blood pressure during exercise or modifying your routine.

Getting Started with Isometrics:

1. Start Slowly: Begin with 2-3 exercises, 1-2 times per week
2. Focus on Form: Proper alignment prevents injury and maximizes benefits
3. Breathe Steadily: Avoid holding your breath during contractions
4. Listen to Your Body: Stop if you experience pain or dizziness

Troubleshooting Tip: If you're unsure about proper form, consider working with a physical therapist or certified senior fitness instructor initially.

Integrating Isometrics into Your Life:

Isometric exercises can be seamlessly incorporated into your daily routine:

1. During TV commercials: Wall sits or doorway presses
2. While waiting in line: Calf raises or glute squeezes
3. At your desk: Abdominal bracing or hand presses

Imagine turning every idle moment into an opportunity for strength building. That's the beauty of isometric exercise for seniors - it fits into your life, rather than disrupting it.

Troubleshooting Tip: Set reminders on your phone or place sticky notes in key areas to prompt you to do quick isometric holds throughout the day.

Remember, isometric exercise is not about pushing to exhaustion or pain. It's about consistent, controlled effort that respects your body's limits while gradually expanding your strength and stability. As we age, this type of exercise becomes invaluable for maintaining independence and quality of life.

In our next section, we'll explore the specific benefits of isometric exercise for seniors in more detail. Are you starting to see how this simple yet powerful form of exercise could fit into your life? Excellent! Let's continue our journey into the world of senior fitness through isometric training.

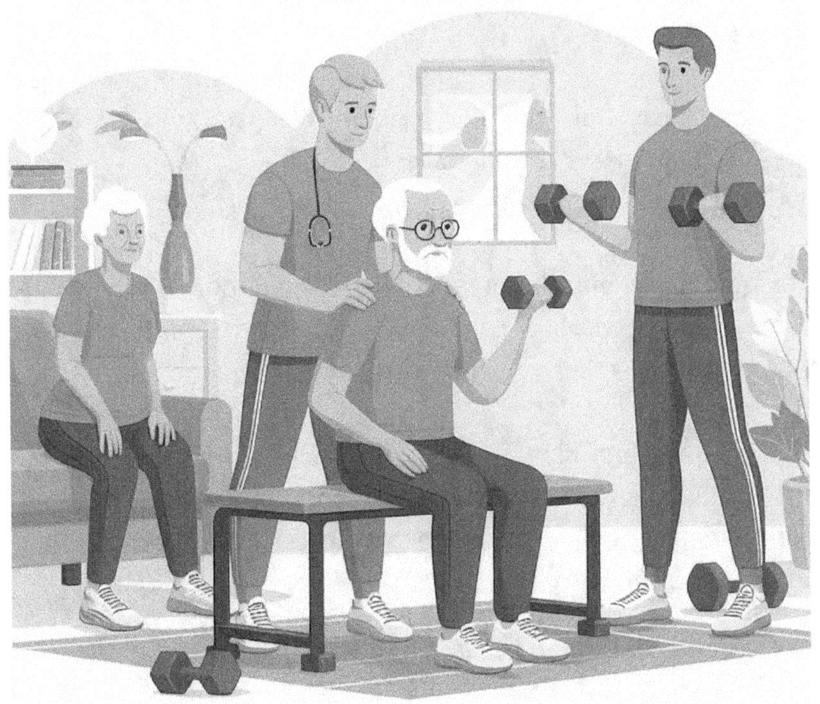

Imagine waking up each morning feeling stronger, more stable, and more confident in your body's abilities. This isn't just a dream - it's the reality that isometric exercises can help create for older adults. Let's explore the numerous benefits that make this form of exercise particularly valuable for seniors.

1. Increased Muscle Strength and Mass

As we age, we naturally lose muscle mass and strength - a condition known as sarcopenia. Isometric exercises can help combat this:

- Maintains and even increases muscle strength
- Helps preserve muscle mass
- Targets specific muscle groups effectively

Imagine your muscles as a strong foundation for a house. Isometric exercises help maintain and reinforce this foundation, keeping your body sturdy and functional.

Troubleshooting Tip: If you're not seeing strength gains, try increasing the intensity of your contractions or holding them for longer periods. Remember, progress might be gradual, but it's significant.

2. Improved Joint Health and Reduced Pain

For many seniors, joint pain can be a significant barrier to exercise. Isometric exercises offer a solution:

- Strengthens muscles around joints without putting stress on the joints themselves
- Can help alleviate pain in conditions like osteoarthritis
- Improves joint stability, potentially reducing the risk of injury

Think of your joints as the hinges on a door. Isometric exercises oil these hinges and strengthen the surrounding structure, making movement smoother and less painful.

Troubleshooting Tip: If you experience increased joint pain during or after isometric exercises, reduce the intensity or duration. Always work within your pain-free range.

3. Enhanced Balance and Fall Prevention

Falls are a major concern for older adults. Isometric exercises can significantly improve balance:

- Strengthens core muscles crucial for stability
- Improves proprioception (your body's sense of position in space)
- Enhances overall body awareness and control

Imagine your body as a ship on the sea. Isometric exercises act like an anchor, providing stability even when the waters get rough.

Troubleshooting Tip: Incorporate balance-specific isometric exercises, like single-leg stands (holding onto a chair for support if needed), to further improve your stability.

4. Cardiovascular Health Benefits

While not a replacement for aerobic exercise, isometric training can benefit heart health:

- May help lower resting blood pressure
- Improves overall cardiovascular endurance
- Can be a safe alternative for those who can't perform traditional cardio exercises

Think of your cardiovascular system as a river. Isometric exercises help strengthen the banks, allowing for better flow and control.

Troubleshooting Tip: Monitor your breathing during isometric holds. If you find yourself holding your breath, focus on maintaining steady, controlled breaths throughout the exercise.

5. Improved Bone Density

Maintaining bone density is crucial for preventing osteoporosis and fractures:

- Isometric exercises create tension in bones, stimulating bone-forming cells
- Can help maintain or even slightly increase bone density
- Particularly beneficial for weight-bearing bones

Imagine your bones as the steel beams in a building. Isometric exercises help keep these beams strong and resistant to wear and tear.

Troubleshooting Tip: Combine isometric exercises with weight-bearing activities (like standing exercises) for maximum bone health benefits.

6. Enhanced Flexibility and Range of Motion

Contrary to what you might think, isometric exercises can improve flexibility:

- Strengthens muscles through their full range of motion
- Can be used to gently stretch tight muscles
- Improves overall mobility when combined with stretching

Think of your muscles as elastic bands. Isometric exercises help maintain their elasticity and prevent them from becoming stiff and rigid.

Troubleshooting Tip: After your isometric routine, spend a few minutes gently stretching the muscles you've worked to maximize flexibility gains.

7. Improved Mental Health and Cognitive Function

The benefits of isometric exercises extend beyond the physical:

- Can reduce symptoms of anxiety and depression
- Improves sleep quality
- May enhance cognitive function and memory

Imagine your brain as a powerful computer. Isometric exercises help keep it running smoothly and efficiently.

Troubleshooting Tip: Try incorporating mindfulness or meditation techniques during your isometric holds to further enhance mental health benefits.

8. Increased Independence and Quality of Life

Perhaps the most significant benefit for older adults is the impact on daily life:

- Improves ability to perform activities of daily living
- Enhances overall energy levels
- Boosts confidence in physical abilities

Think of isometric exercises as a key that unlocks a more active, independent lifestyle.

Troubleshooting Tip: Set small, achievable goals related to daily activities (like easily getting up from a chair) to track your progress and stay motivated.

9. Low Risk of Injury

Compared to many other forms of exercise, isometrics offer a safer alternative:

- No dynamic movements that could cause falls
- Minimal joint stress
- Easily modifiable to individual fitness levels

Imagine isometric exercises as a gentle yet effective way to nurture your body, minimizing risks while maximizing benefits.

Troubleshooting Tip: Always start with a lower intensity and gradually increase as you become more comfortable with the exercises.

10. Convenience and Accessibility

One of the greatest advantages of isometric exercises for seniors is their practicality:

- Can be done anywhere, anytime
- Requires no special equipment
- Easily incorporated into daily routines

Think of isometric exercises as a portable gym that you carry with you wherever you go.

Troubleshooting Tip: Create an "isometric exercise menu" with quick exercises you can do in various situations (waiting in line, watching TV, etc.) to make it easier to incorporate them into your day.

Remember, the key to reaping these benefits is consistency and proper form. In our next section, we'll discuss important safety considerations to ensure you can enjoy these benefits without risk. Are you excited to start experiencing these benefits for yourself? Great! Let's continue our journey into the world of isometric exercise for seniors.

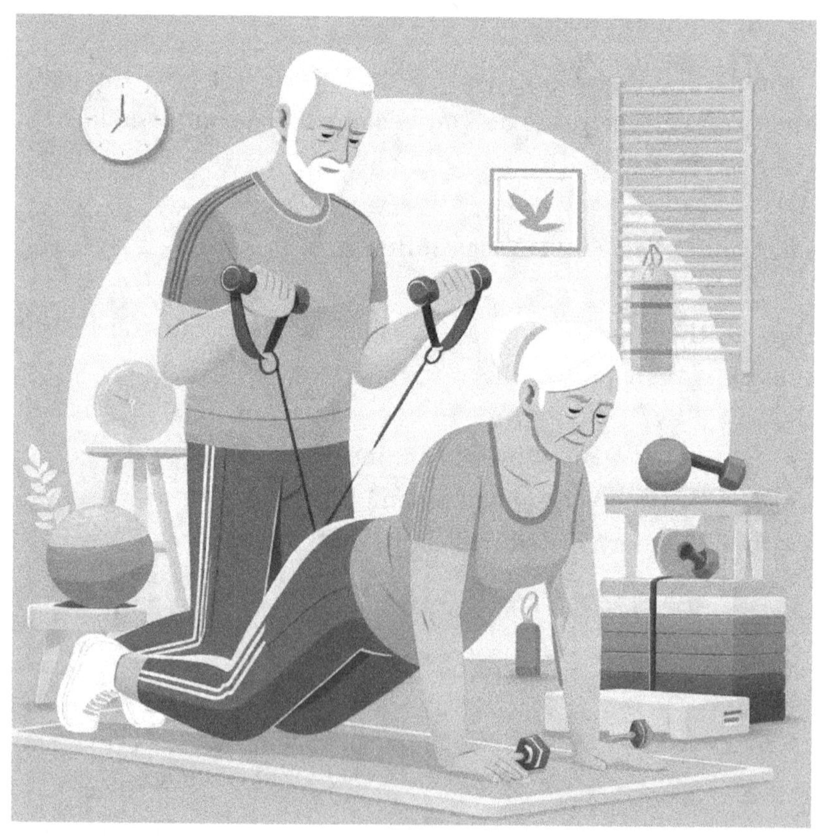

Imagine embarking on a journey to better health and strength. Like any journey, it's crucial to have a map and know the potential pitfalls. That's what these safety considerations are - your guide to practicing isometric exercises safely and effectively.

1. Consult Your Healthcare Provider

Before starting any new exercise regimen, it's crucial to get the green light from your doctor.

Why it's important:
- Ensures exercises are safe for your specific health conditions
- Helps identify any necessary modifications
- Can provide valuable insights into your physical capabilities

Think of your doctor as the expert navigator on your fitness journey, helping you chart the safest and most effective course.

Troubleshooting Tip: Prepare a list of questions about isometric exercises and your health conditions before your appointment to ensure a productive discussion.

2. Start Slowly and Progress Gradually

Patience is key when beginning isometric exercises.

Key points:
- Begin with shorter hold times (5-10 seconds)
- Start with 1-2 exercises per muscle group
- Gradually increase duration, intensity, and frequency

Imagine your fitness journey as climbing a staircase. It's much safer and more effective to take one step at a time rather than trying to leap to the top.

Troubleshooting Tip: Keep a log of your exercises, including hold times and perceived effort. This can help you track progress and ensure you're advancing at a safe pace.

3. Maintain Proper Form

Correct technique is crucial for both safety and effectiveness.

Why it's important:
- Prevents strain on joints and muscles
- Ensures targeted muscles are engaged correctly
- Maximizes benefits of the exercises

Think of proper form as the foundation of a building. Without it, the entire structure is at risk.

Troubleshooting Tip: Use a mirror when starting out to check your form, or consider working with a physical therapist or certified fitness instructor initially to ensure you're performing exercises correctly.

4. Listen to Your Body

Pain is your body's way of signaling that something isn't right.

Key points:
- Distinguish between muscle fatigue and pain
- Stop if you experience sharp or sudden pain
- Be aware of any dizziness or shortness of breath

Imagine your body as a finely tuned instrument. Learning to interpret its signals is crucial for safe exercise.

Troubleshooting Tip: Develop a pain scale from 1-10. If pain exceeds a 3 or 4 during exercise, stop and reassess your technique or the exercise itself.

5. Breathe Properly

Proper breathing technique is often overlooked but is crucial for safety.

Why it's important:
- Prevents unnecessary increase in blood pressure
- Ensures adequate oxygen supply to muscles
- Helps maintain stability during holds

Think of your breath as the rhythm section in a band, providing a steady beat for your exercise routine.

Troubleshooting Tip: Practice breathing slowly and steadily through your nose during holds. If you find yourself holding your breath, reduce the intensity of the contraction.

6. Be Mindful of Blood Pressure

Isometric exercises can cause a temporary increase in blood pressure.

Key considerations:
- Particularly important for those with hypertension
- Avoid holding breath during contractions
- Monitor how you feel during and after exercises

Imagine your cardiovascular system as a network of pipes. Proper technique helps manage the pressure in these pipes during exercise.

Troubleshooting Tip: If you have hypertension, consider using a home blood pressure monitor to check your readings before and after your exercise sessions.

7. Use Support When Needed

Don't hesitate to use chairs, walls, or other stable objects for support.

Why it's important:
- Prevents falls and injuries
- Allows you to focus on the exercise rather than balance
- Provides confidence to try new exercises

Think of these supports as your safety harness, allowing you to challenge yourself while minimizing risk.

Troubleshooting Tip: Ensure any object you're using for support is stable. A sturdy chair is often better than a less stable object like a table.

8. Stay Hydrated

Proper hydration is crucial, even though isometric exercises may not feel as intense as other forms of exercise.

Key points:
- Drink water before, during, and after your exercise session
- Be aware of increased need for hydration in warmer environments
- Watch for signs of dehydration (dizziness, dry mouth, dark urine)

Imagine your body as a plant. Regular watering keeps it healthy and functioning optimally.

Troubleshooting Tip: Keep a water bottle visible during your exercise routine as a reminder to drink regularly.

9. Warm Up and Cool Down

Preparing your body for exercise and allowing it to recover is crucial.

Why it's important:
- Warms up muscles and increases flexibility
- Gradually raises heart rate
- Helps prevent injury and reduces post-exercise soreness

Think of your warm-up and cool-down as the prelude and epilogue to a great story - they set the stage and help you transition smoothly.

Troubleshooting Tip: Include gentle stretches and low-intensity movements in your warm-up and cool-down routines.

10. Be Aware of Your Environment

Ensure your exercise space is safe and free from hazards.

Key considerations:
- Remove tripping hazards
- Ensure adequate lighting
- Have a sturdy chair or wall nearby for support if needed

Imagine your exercise space as your personal safety zone. Taking time to set it up properly can prevent accidents.

Troubleshooting Tip: Do a quick "safety scan" of your exercise area before each session, looking for potential hazards.

11. Listen to Your Healthcare Provider's Advice

If you have specific health conditions, follow your doctor's recommendations closely.

Key points:
- Adhere to any exercise restrictions
- Be aware of warning signs specific to your condition
- Regular check-ins with your healthcare provider can help monitor progress and adjust as needed

Think of your healthcare provider's advice as a personalized roadmap for your fitness journey.

Troubleshooting Tip: Keep a list of any exercise restrictions or special considerations from your doctor in your exercise area as a reminder.

Remember, safety is the foundation of an effective exercise routine. By following these guidelines, you're setting yourself up for a successful and beneficial isometric exercise practice. In our next section, we'll explore how to assess your current fitness level and set realistic goals. Are you feeling more confident about exercising safely? Excellent! Let's continue our journey into the world of isometric exercise for seniors.

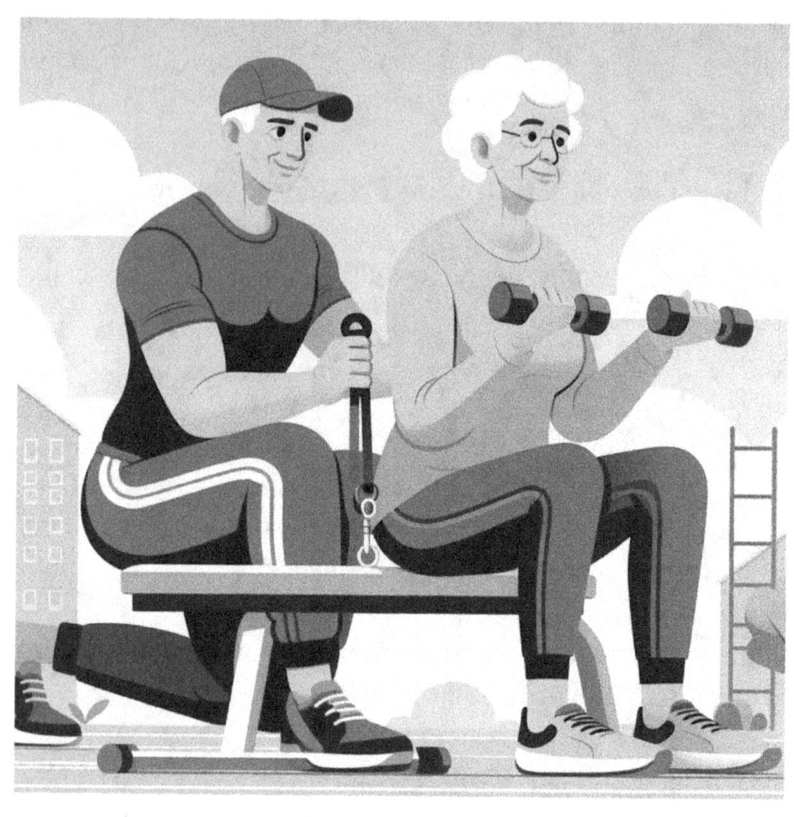

Imagine you're about to embark on a journey. Before setting out, you'd want to know where you're starting from, right? That's exactly what assessing your fitness level is all about. It's your starting point on the map of your isometric exercise journey.

Why Assessing Your Fitness Level is Important:

- Provides a baseline to measure progress
- Helps identify areas that need more focus
- Ensures you start at an appropriate level
- Allows for personalized goal setting

Think of this assessment as taking a snapshot of your current physical condition. It's not about judgment, but about understanding where you are so you can plan where you want to go.

Key Areas to Assess:

1. Muscular Strength

This refers to how much force your muscles can produce.

How to assess:
- Wall push test: How long can you hold a wall push?
- Chair stand test: How many times can you stand up from a chair in 30 seconds?

Troubleshooting Tip: If you can't perform these tests fully, modify them. For example, do wall pushes at an angle or use your arms to assist in standing from the chair. The goal is to get a baseline, not to strain yourself.

2. Muscular Endurance

This is about how long your muscles can sustain an activity.

How to assess:
- Plank hold: How long can you hold a plank position (on knees if needed)?
- Wall sit: How long can you hold a wall sit?

Troubleshooting Tip: Use a timer and stop when you feel significant fatigue, not when you're completely exhausted. Safety first!

3. Flexibility

Flexibility is crucial for maintaining range of motion and preventing injury.

How to assess:
- Sit and reach test: Sitting on the floor, how far can you reach towards your toes?

- Shoulder flexibility test: Can you reach behind your back and touch your shoulder blades?

Troubleshooting Tip: Don't force any stretches. The point is to assess your current flexibility, not to increase it immediately.

4. Balance

Good balance is essential for preventing falls and maintaining independence.

How to assess:
- Single leg stand: How long can you stand on one leg (use a chair for support if needed)?
- Tandem stand: Can you stand heel-to-toe for 10 seconds?

Troubleshooting Tip: Always have a stable support nearby when testing balance. Safety is paramount.

5. Cardiovascular Endurance

While isometric exercises aren't primarily cardio, it's good to know your baseline.

How to assess:
- 2-minute step test: How many times can you raise your knees to a marked point on the wall in 2 minutes?

Troubleshooting Tip: If you can't do the full 2 minutes, that's okay. Note how long you could go and use that as your baseline.

6. Body Composition

While not directly related to isometric exercise, it's a good overall health indicator.

How to assess:
- Body Mass Index (BMI): Use a BMI calculator
- Waist circumference: Measure your waist at the navel

Troubleshooting Tip: Remember, these are just numbers. They don't define you or your fitness journey.

How to Conduct Your Assessment:

1. Choose a time when you're well-rested and not immediately after a meal.
2. Warm up gently before starting.
3. Have someone present to assist and ensure safety, if possible.
4. Record your results in a journal or fitness app.
5. Be honest with yourself - this is your starting point, not a competition.

Troubleshooting Tip: If you're uncomfortable with any part of the assessment, skip it. You can always come back to it later when you feel more confident.

Interpreting Your Results:

Remember, these assessments are personal benchmarks, not competitions. Compare your results to standardized charts for your age group if available, but more importantly, use them as your own baseline for future comparison.

Imagine these results as the first page in your fitness story. They're just the beginning, and the most exciting chapters are yet to come.

Next Steps:

1. Share your results with your healthcare provider or a fitness professional.
2. Use these results to set realistic, achievable goals.
3. Plan to reassess every 4-6 weeks to track progress.

Troubleshooting Tip: If you're discouraged by your initial results, remember: every fitness journey starts somewhere. The fact that you're assessing yourself is already a big step forward!

Remember, assessing your fitness level isn't about judgment. It's about understanding where you are so you can celebrate your progress as you move forward. In our next section, we'll discuss how to use these results to set realistic and achievable goals for your isometric exercise journey.

Are you feeling more aware of your current fitness level? Excellent! This self-awareness is the first step towards a stronger, healthier you. Let's continue our exploration of isometric exercise for seniors.

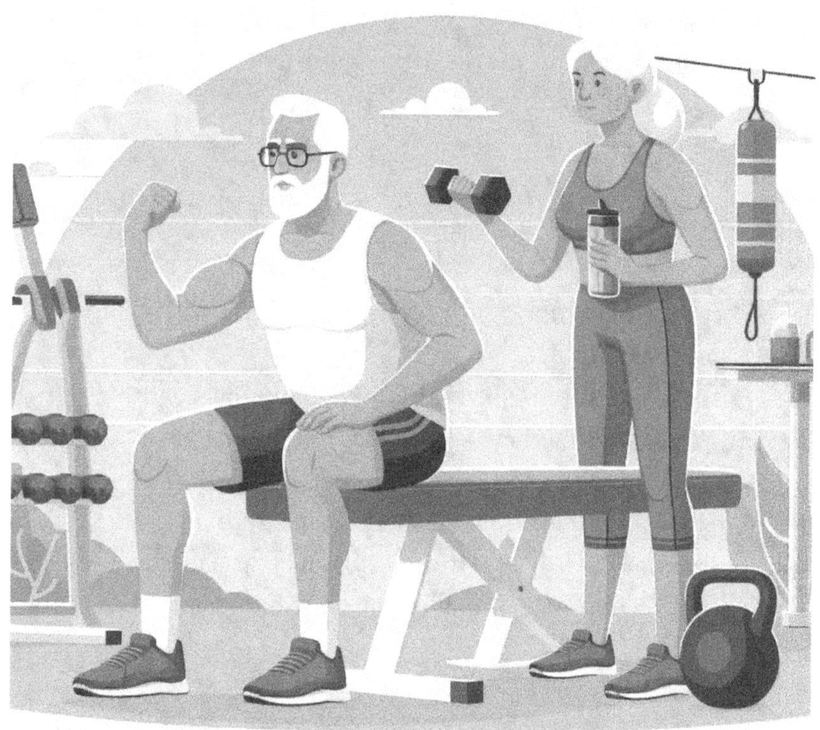

Imagine you're planning a trip to a destination you've never visited before. You wouldn't just start walking without a map or a plan, would you? Setting realistic goals is like creating your personal roadmap for your fitness journey. It gives you direction, motivation, and a way to measure your progress.

Why Setting Realistic Goals is Crucial:

- Provides clear direction for your efforts
- Keeps you motivated and engaged
- Allows you to track progress and celebrate achievements
- Helps prevent frustration and burnout

Think of your goals as the stepping stones across a river. Each one gets you closer to the other side, but they need to be placed at reachable distances to ensure a safe crossing.

Key Principles for Setting Realistic Goals:

1. Be Specific

Vague goals like "get stronger" are hard to measure. Instead, aim for specificity.

Examples:
- "Hold a wall sit for 30 seconds"
- "Perform 10 chair stands without using my arms"

Troubleshooting Tip: If you're struggling to be specific, think about daily activities you'd like to improve. For instance, "Climb stairs without getting winded" is a specific, functional goal.

2. Make it Measurable

Your goals should be quantifiable so you can track progress.

Examples:
- "Increase plank hold time by 5 seconds each week"
- "Improve balance to stand on one foot for 20 seconds"

Troubleshooting Tip: Use a journal or fitness app to record your measurements. Seeing the numbers improve over time can be incredibly motivating.

3. Ensure it's Achievable

While it's good to challenge yourself, setting impossible goals can lead to discouragement.

Examples:
- If you currently can't do a wall push-up, aim to hold the position for 5 seconds first, before progressing to a full push-up
- If standing from a chair is difficult, start with a higher chair and gradually lower the height

Troubleshooting Tip: Break larger goals into smaller, manageable steps. Each small achievement will boost your confidence and keep you moving forward.

4. Make it Relevant

Your goals should align with your overall health and lifestyle objectives.

Examples:
- If fall prevention is a concern, focus on balance and leg strength goals
- If you want to play with grandchildren, set goals related to endurance and flexibility

Troubleshooting Tip: Regularly remind yourself why these goals matter to you. Connecting your exercises to real-life benefits can boost motivation.

5. Set a Timeframe

Having a timeline creates a sense of urgency and helps you stay on track.

Examples:
- "Perform a 30-second wall sit by the end of the month"
- "Increase my plank hold time to 1 minute within 8 weeks"

Troubleshooting Tip: Be flexible with your timelines. If you don't meet a goal by the set date, don't get discouraged. Adjust the timeline or break the goal into smaller steps.

Types of Goals to Consider:

1. Strength Goals
Focus on increasing the duration or intensity of isometric holds.

Example: "Hold a doorway chest press for 15 seconds by the end of the month"

2. Endurance Goals
Aim to increase the number of repetitions or sets you can perform.

Example: "Complete 3 sets of 10-second isometric bicep curls within 6 weeks"

3. Flexibility Goals
Target improved range of motion through isometric stretching.

Example: "Touch my toes while sitting (and hold for 10 seconds) within 2 months"

4. Functional Goals
Connect your isometric training to daily activities.

Example: "Carry groceries from the car to the house without needing to rest within 3 months"

5. Consistency Goals
Focus on establishing a regular exercise routine.

Example: "Perform isometric exercises for 15 minutes, 3 times a week for the next month"

Troubleshooting Tip: Start with 2-3 goals across different categories. This provides a balanced approach to your fitness journey.

How to Set Your Goals:

1. Reflect on Your Assessment: Use your fitness assessment results as a starting point.

2. Identify Areas for Improvement: Choose areas where you'd like to see progress.

3. Consider Your Motivations: Think about why you're starting this journey.

4. Be Realistic: Set goals that challenge you but are achievable with consistent effort.

5. Write Them Down: Put your goals in writing and place them somewhere visible.

6. Share Your Goals: Tell a friend or family member who can offer support and accountability.

Troubleshooting Tip: If you're unsure about appropriate goals, consult with a physical therapist or certified fitness instructor who specializes in senior fitness.

Adjusting Your Goals:

Remember, goal-setting is not a one-time event. As you progress in your isometric training:

- Regularly review your goals (every 4-6 weeks is a good interval)
- Celebrate achievements, no matter how small
- Adjust goals that seem too easy or too challenging
- Add new goals as you accomplish existing ones

Think of your goals as a living document, evolving as you grow stronger and more confident in your abilities.

Troubleshooting Tip: If you find yourself consistently missing your goals, it's time to reassess. There's no shame in adjusting – the important thing is to keep moving forward.

Remember, the journey of isometric exercise is personal and unique to you. Your goals should reflect your individual needs, desires, and capabilities. By setting realistic, achievable goals, you're setting yourself up for success and a more fulfilling fitness journey.

In our next section, we'll discuss creating a workout schedule that aligns with your goals and fits into your lifestyle. Are you feeling inspired to set some personal fitness goals? Fantastic! Let's continue our exploration of isometric exercise for seniors.

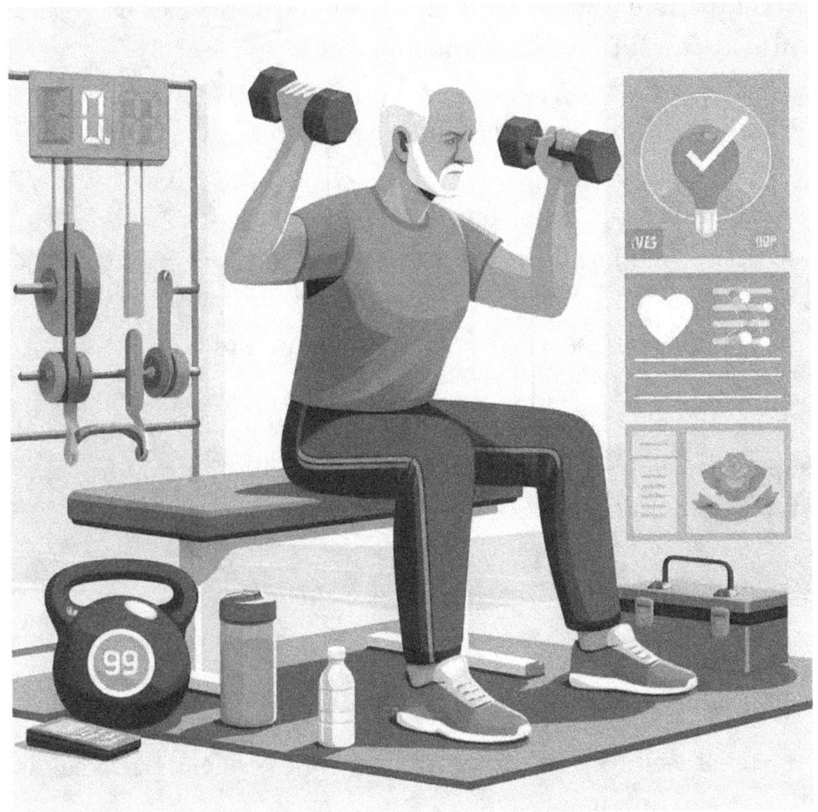

Imagine you're tending a garden. You wouldn't water it sporadically and expect it to thrive, would you? Similarly, a consistent workout schedule is the key to nurturing your strength and health through isometric exercises. Let's cultivate a routine that works for you.

Why a Workout Schedule is Important:

- Establishes a consistent routine
- Helps balance different muscle groups
- Ensures adequate rest and recovery
- Makes exercise a habit, not an afterthought

Think of your workout schedule as the scaffolding that supports your fitness goals. It provides structure and stability to your efforts.

Key Principles for Creating Your Schedule:

1. Frequency

For most seniors, 2-3 isometric workout sessions per week is a good starting point.

Why it matters:
- Allows for adequate recovery between sessions
- Frequent enough to see progress
- Helps establish a consistent routine

Troubleshooting Tip: If 2-3 full sessions seem daunting, start with shorter, more frequent sessions. Even 5-10 minutes daily can be beneficial.

2. Duration

Aim for 15-30 minutes per session, depending on your current fitness level.

Why it matters:
- Long enough to provide benefits
- Short enough to fit into busy schedules
- Prevents fatigue and overexertion

Troubleshooting Tip: If 15 minutes feels too long, break it into two 7-8 minute sessions throughout the day.

3. Timing

Choose times when you typically have the most energy and fewest distractions.

Why it matters:
- Increases likelihood of sticking to the schedule
- Helps you perform exercises with better focus and form

Troubleshooting Tip: Experiment with different times of day to find what works best for you. Some people prefer mornings, others find afternoon or evening workouts more enjoyable.

4. Balance

Ensure your schedule includes exercises for all major muscle groups.

Why it matters:
- Prevents muscle imbalances
- Provides comprehensive strength benefits
- Supports overall functional fitness

Troubleshooting Tip: Use a checklist to ensure you're targeting all major muscle groups over the course of your weekly routine.

5. Progression

Plan to gradually increase the duration or intensity of your workouts over time.

Why it matters:
- Allows for continuous improvement
- Prevents plateaus in strength gains
- Keeps the routine challenging and engaging

Troubleshooting Tip: Aim to increase either the duration of holds or the number of repetitions by about 10% every 1-2 weeks.

Sample Weekly Schedule:

Monday:
- 20-minute session focusing on lower body and core
- Examples: Wall sits, standing calf raises, abdominal bracing

Wednesday:
- 20-minute session focusing on upper body and balance
- Examples: Doorway chest press, wall push-ups, single-leg stands

Friday:
- 20-minute full-body session
- Examples: Plank holds, isometric lunges, overhead press against a wall

Troubleshooting Tip: Always include a 5-minute warm-up and cool-down in your sessions. This can be as simple as marching in place and gentle stretching.

Integrating Isometrics into Daily Life:

Beyond scheduled workouts, look for opportunities to incorporate isometric exercises into your daily routine:

- Hold a squat while brushing your teeth
- Do calf raises while waiting in line
- Practice hand squeezes while watching TV

Think of these as "exercise snacks" - small doses of strength work that add up over time.

Troubleshooting Tip: Set reminders on your phone or place sticky notes around your home to prompt these "exercise snacks."

Adapting Your Schedule:

Remember, flexibility is key. Your schedule should adapt to your life, not the other way around.

Consider:
- Seasonal changes (e.g., outdoor exercises in good weather)
- Health fluctuations (e.g., lighter workouts during recovery from illness)
- Social commitments (e.g., adjusting workout times around family visits)

Troubleshooting Tip: Have a "Plan B" workout ready - a shorter routine you can fall back on when time is tight or energy is low.

Tracking Your Schedule:

Use a method that works for you to keep track of your workouts:
- A paper calendar
- A fitness app
- A journal

Why it matters:
- Provides accountability
- Allows you to see patterns in your routine
- Gives a sense of accomplishment as you check off completed workouts

Troubleshooting Tip: Reward yourself for consistency. Maybe treat yourself to something special after a month of sticking to your schedule.

Listen to Your Body:

While consistency is important, it's crucial to respect your body's signals:
- If you're feeling unusually fatigued, it's okay to take an extra rest day
- If you're feeling energized, it's fine to add an extra short session

Think of your body as a wise advisor. Learn to listen to its feedback and adjust accordingly.

Troubleshooting Tip: Keep a log of how you feel before and after each workout. This can help you identify patterns and optimize your schedule over time.

Remember, the best workout schedule is one that you can stick to consistently. It should challenge you without overwhelming you, fit into your life without dominating it, and most importantly, be enjoyable.

In our next section, we'll dive into specific upper body isometric exercises. Are you feeling ready to create your personal isometric workout schedule? Excellent! Let's continue our journey into the world of isometric exercise for seniors.

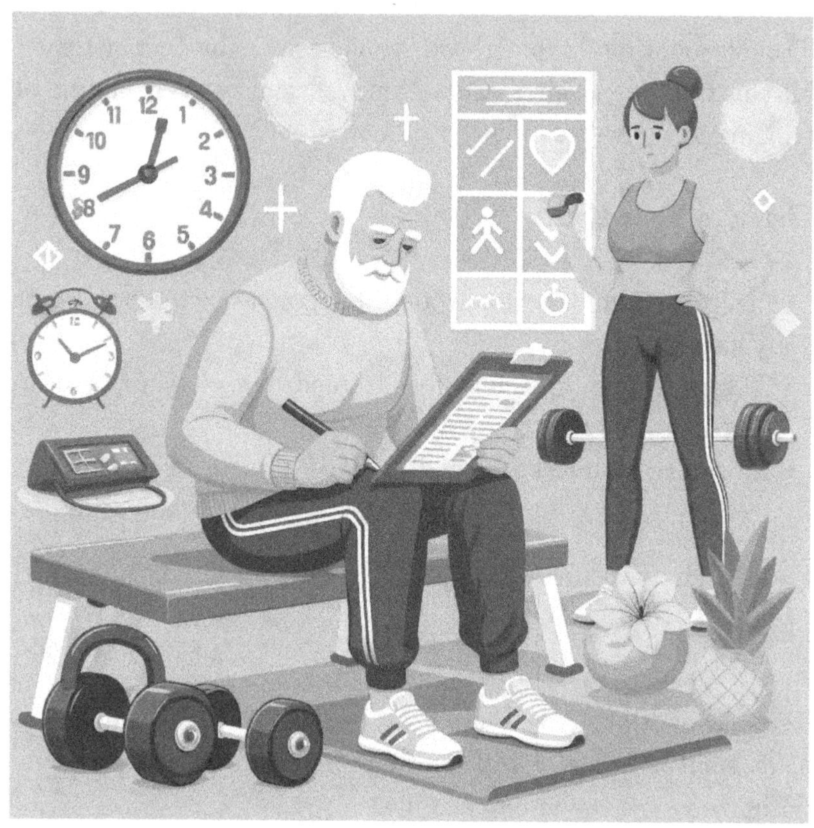

Shoulder and neck exercises

Imagine your shoulders and neck as the control tower of your upper body. Keeping them strong and flexible is crucial for many daily activities, from reaching for objects to maintaining good posture. Let's explore some isometric exercises that can help strengthen this important area.

1. Wall Press for Shoulders

This exercise targets your shoulder muscles and upper chest.

Steps:
1. Stand facing a wall, about an arm's length away.
2. Place your palms flat against the wall at shoulder height, shoulder-width apart.
3. Lean in slightly, keeping your body straight from head to heels.
4. Push against the wall as if you're trying to move it.
5. Hold this position for 10-15 seconds while breathing normally.
6. Relax and repeat 3-5 times.

Troubleshooting Tip: If you feel any strain in your lower back, take a small step closer to the wall and ensure your core is engaged.

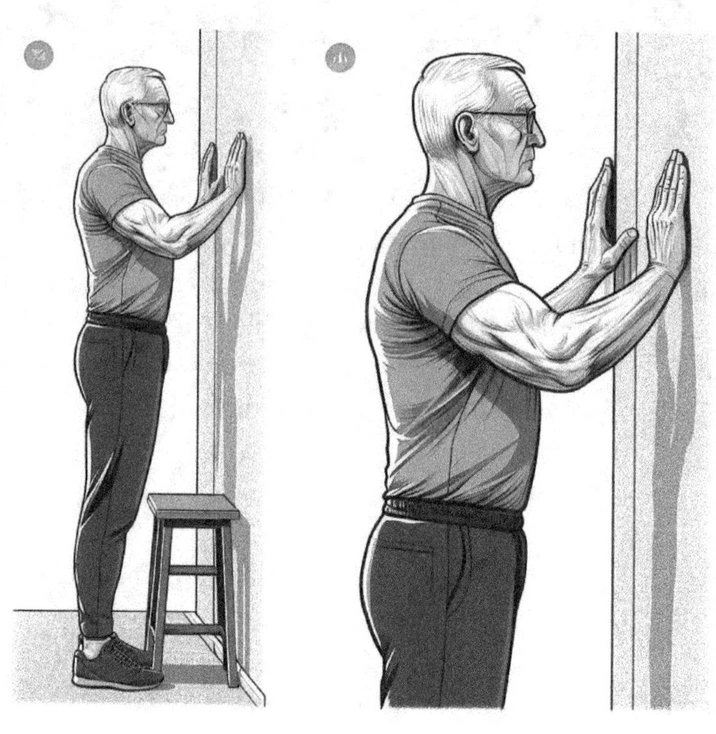

2. Neck Press

This exercise strengthens the muscles in your neck.

Steps:
1. Sit comfortably in a chair with your back straight.
2. Place your right hand on the right side of your head, above your ear.
3. Gently press your head into your hand while keeping your head straight.
4. Resist the movement with your hand so your head doesn't actually tilt.
5. Hold for 5-10 seconds, then relax.
6. Repeat on the left side.
7. Do 3-5 repetitions on each side.

Troubleshooting Tip: If you experience any dizziness or discomfort, reduce the pressure or consult with your healthcare provider before continuing.

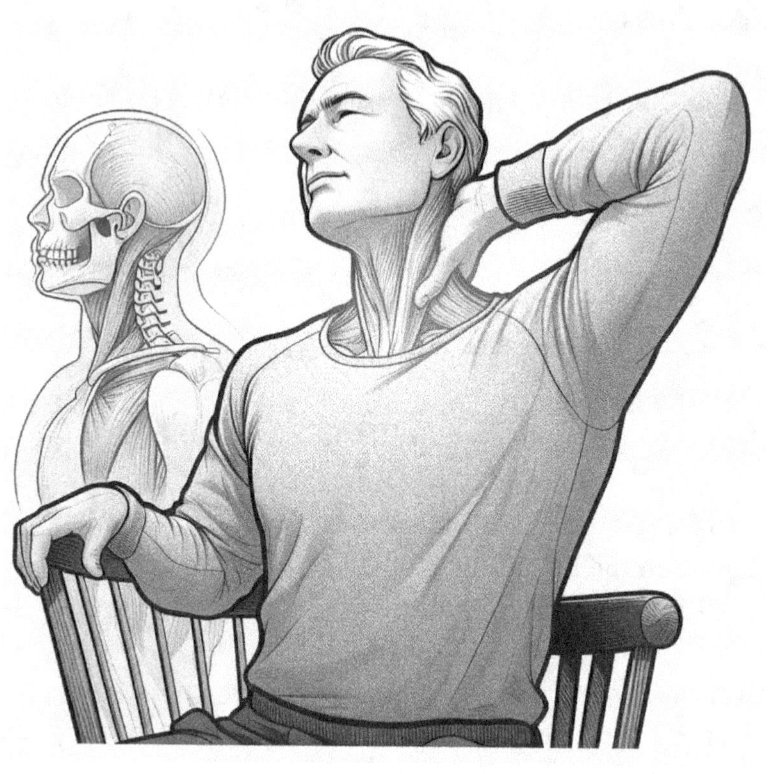

3. Shoulder Blade Squeeze

This exercise improves posture and strengthens the muscles between your shoulder blades.

Steps:
1. Sit or stand with your arms relaxed at your sides.
2. Slowly squeeze your shoulder blades together, as if trying to hold a pencil between them.
3. Hold this position for 5-10 seconds.
4. Slowly relax.
5. Repeat 5-8 times.

Troubleshooting Tip: Focus on using your back muscles, not your arms. If you feel tension in your arms, shake them out and try again with less intensity.

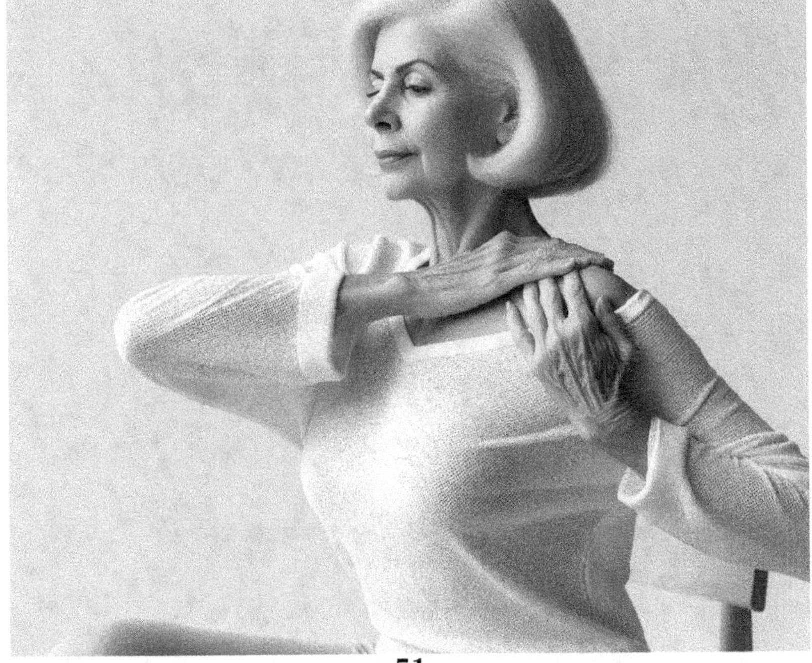

4. Overhead Press

This exercise targets your shoulder muscles and upper arms.

Steps:
1. Stand facing a wall, about an arm's length away.
2. Raise your arms and place your palms flat against the wall at about head height.
3. Press upward against the wall as if trying to push the ceiling up.
4. Hold for 10-15 seconds while breathing normally.
5. Relax and repeat 3-5 times.

Troubleshooting Tip: If reaching overhead is uncomfortable, lower your hands to a position that feels comfortable and work on gradually raising them over time.

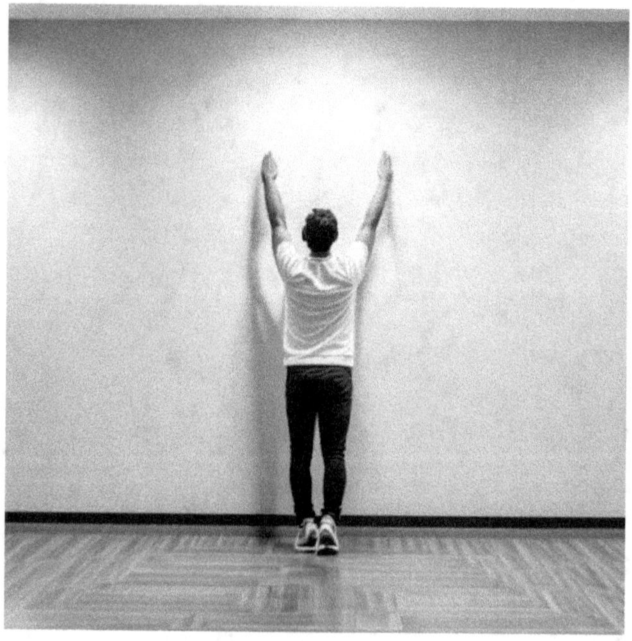

5. Chin Tuck

This exercise helps improve neck posture and can alleviate tension.

Steps:
1. Sit or stand with your back straight.
2. Without tilting your head, gently draw your chin back, creating a "double chin."
3. Hold this position for 5-10 seconds.
4. Relax and repeat 5-8 times.

Troubleshooting Tip: Imagine you're holding an egg between your chin and chest to avoid pressing too hard.

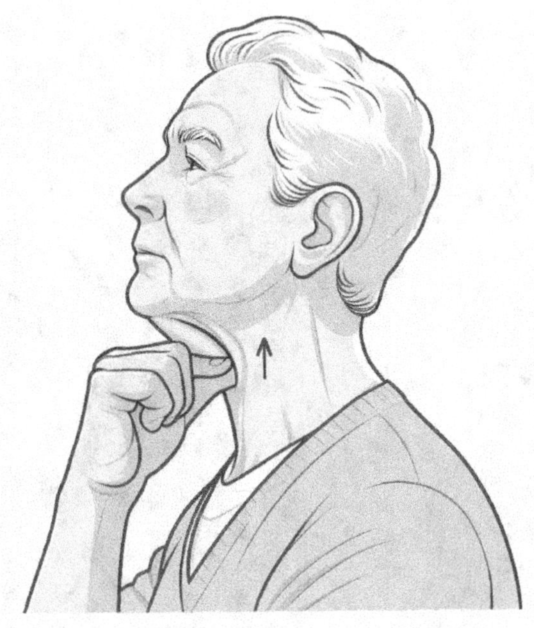

6. Shoulder Shrug

This exercise targets the upper trapezius muscles, which can help relieve neck tension.

Steps:
1. Stand or sit with your arms at your sides.
2. Slowly raise your shoulders towards your ears as high as you comfortably can.
3. Hold this "shrugged" position for 5-10 seconds.
4. Slowly lower your shoulders back down.
5. Repeat 5-8 times.

Troubleshooting Tip: If you feel any pinching or sharp pain, reduce the height of your shrug or consult with a healthcare provider.

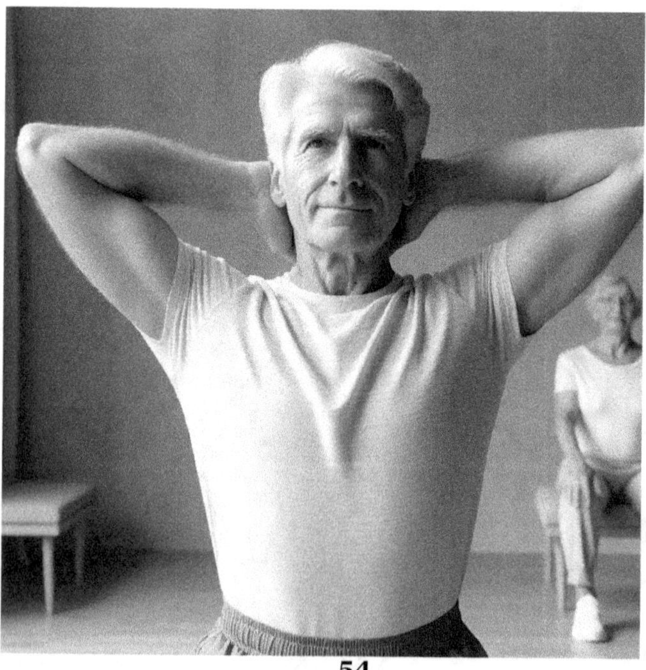

7. Doorway Shoulder Stretch

While not strictly isometric, this stretch can help improve shoulder flexibility.

Steps:
1. Stand in an open doorway.
2. Raise your arms to the sides, bent at a 90-degree angle (like a goal post).
3. Place your palms on the door frame.
4. Slowly lean forward until you feel a gentle stretch in your chest and shoulders.

5. Hold for 15-30 seconds while breathing deeply.
6. Slowly return to the starting position.
7. Repeat 2-3 times.

Troubleshooting Tip: If you can't comfortably reach the top of the door frame, lower your arms to a comfortable height.

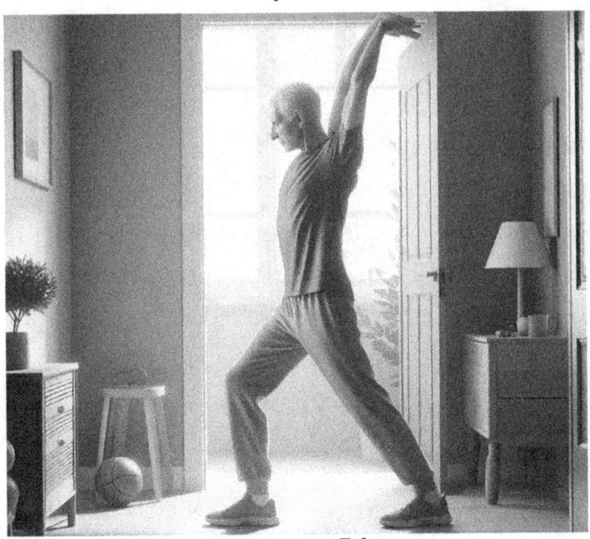

General Tips for Shoulder and Neck Exercises:

1. Warm-up: Always start with gentle neck rolls and shoulder circles to warm up the area.
2. Breathe: Remember to breathe normally throughout each exercise.
3. Stay within your comfort zone: Never push to the point of pain.
4. Consistency is key: Aim to perform these exercises 2-3 times per week.
5. Progressive overload: Gradually increase hold times as you get stronger.

Troubleshooting Tip: If you experience any persistent pain or discomfort during or after these exercises, consult with a healthcare provider or a physical therapist.

Remember, the goal of these exercises is to build strength and improve flexibility gradually. It's not about pushing to your limits, but about consistent, mindful practice. As you incorporate these exercises into your routine, you may notice improved posture, reduced neck tension, and greater ease in daily activities involving your upper body.

In our next section, we'll explore isometric exercises for the arms and chest. Are you feeling ready to give these shoulder and neck exercises a try? Excellent! Let's continue our journey into the world of isometric exercise for seniors.

Imagine your arms and chest as the powerhouse of your upper body. Strengthening these areas can make daily activities like carrying groceries, opening jars, or pushing doors much easier. Let's dive into some effective isometric exercises for your arms and chest.

1. Wall Push

This exercise targets your chest, shoulders, and triceps.

Steps:
1. Stand facing a wall, about arm's length away.
2. Place your palms flat on the wall at chest height, slightly wider than shoulder-width apart.
3. Lean in, bending your elbows slightly.
4. Push against the wall as if trying to move it.
5. Hold this position for 10-15 seconds while breathing normally.
6. Relax and repeat 3-5 times.

Troubleshooting Tip: If you feel strain in your wrists, try forming a fist and pushing with your knuckles instead.

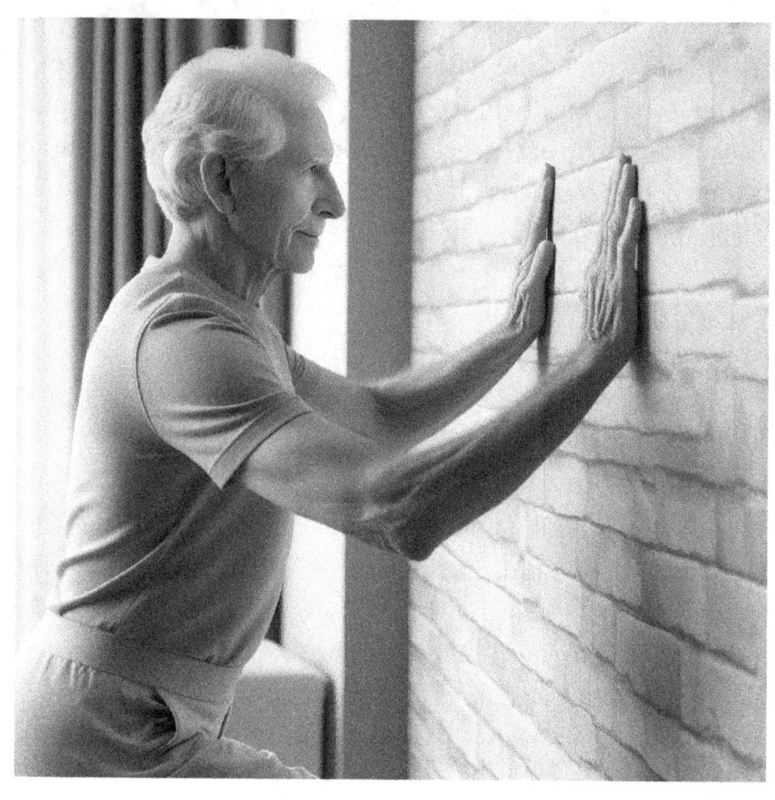

2. Doorway Chest Press

This exercise focuses on your chest muscles and biceps.

Steps:
1. Stand in an open doorway.
2. Raise your arms to the sides, bent at a 90-degree angle.
3. Place your forearms on either side of the doorframe.
4. Gently press outward against the frame.
5. Hold for 10-15 seconds, breathing steadily.
6. Relax and repeat 3-5 times.

Troubleshooting Tip: If reaching this height is uncomfortable, lower your arms to a position that feels comfortable and work on gradually raising them over time.

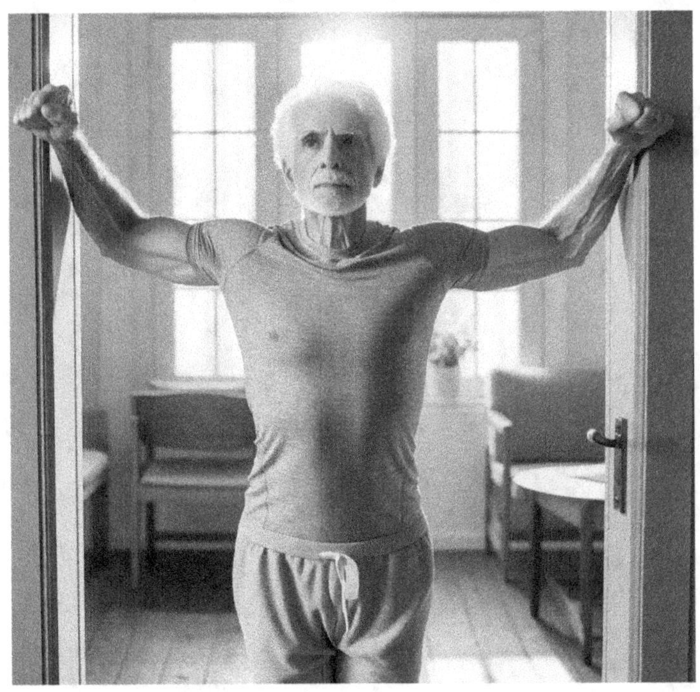

3. Isometric Bicep Curl

This exercise targets your biceps.

Steps:
1. Sit in a sturdy chair with armrests.
2. Place your hands under the armrests, palms facing up.
3. Try to curl your arms upward, but resist the movement with the chair.
4. Hold this position for 10-15 seconds.
5. Relax and repeat 3-5 times.

Troubleshooting Tip: If you don't have a chair with armrests, try pressing your palms together in front of your chest instead.

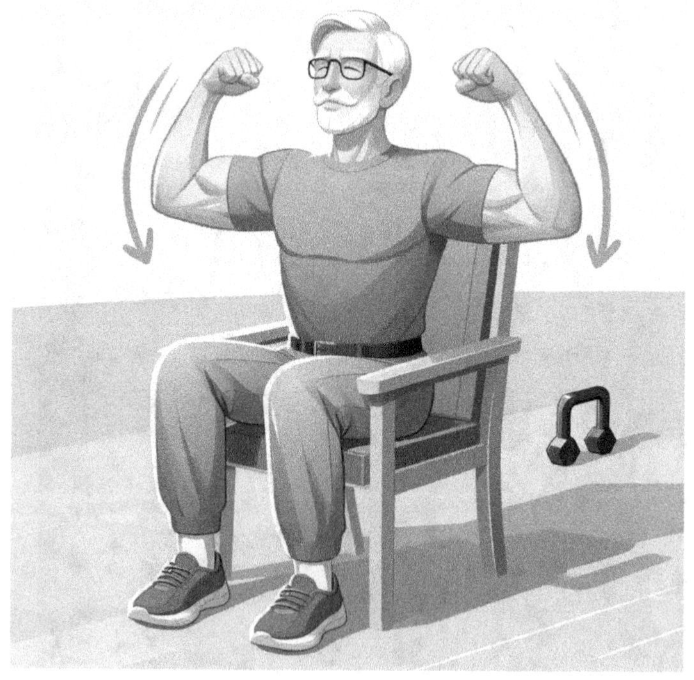

4. Table Press for Triceps

This exercise works your triceps, the muscles at the back of
your upper arms.
Steps:
1. Sit at a table with your hands resting on the edge, palms
down.
2. Slide your bottom forward slightly in the chair.
3. Push down on the table as if trying to lift yourself.
4. Hold for 10-15 seconds while keeping your feet on the
ground.
5. Relax and repeat 3-5 times.

Troubleshooting Tip: If this is too intense, start by just
pressing lightly and gradually increase the pressure as you
get stronger.

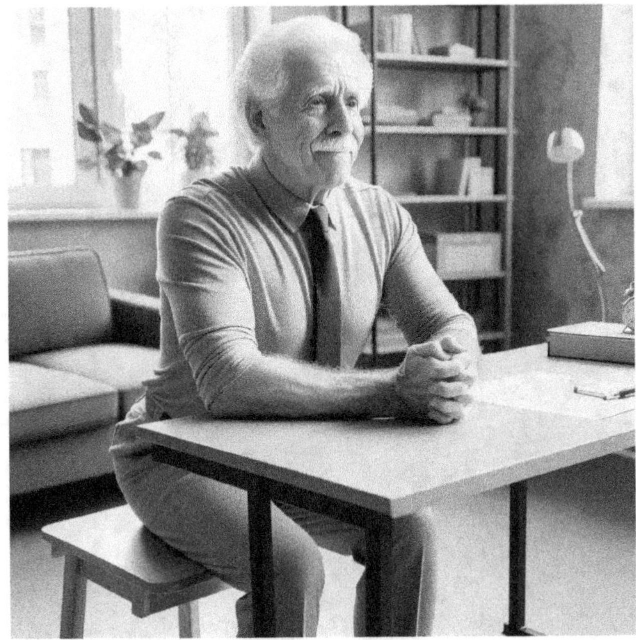

5. Palm Press for Forearms

This exercise strengthens your forearms and improves grip strength.

Steps:
1. Sit comfortably with your elbows resting on a table.
2. Press your palms together in front of your chest, fingers pointing upward.
3. Push your hands against each other with moderate pressure.
4. Hold for 10-15 seconds.
5. Relax and repeat 3-5 times.

Troubleshooting Tip: If you feel any wrist discomfort, try lowering your hands slightly or reducing the pressure.

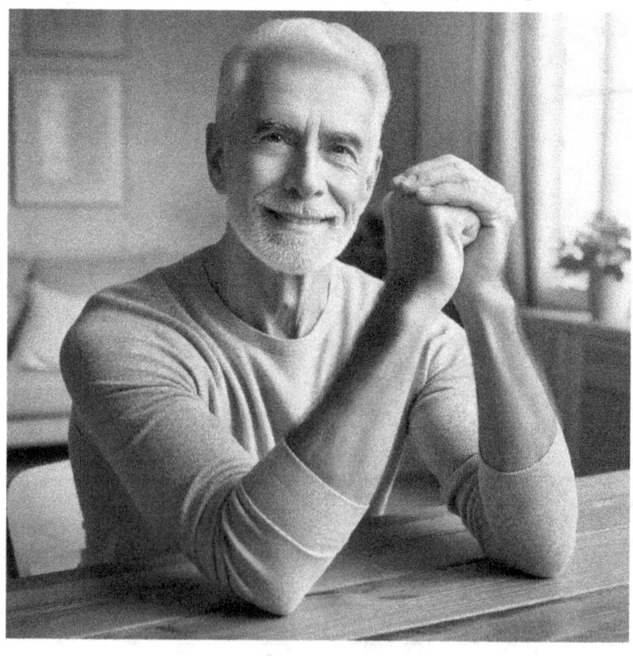

6. Imaginary Box Hold

This exercise works multiple arm muscles simultaneously.

Steps:
1. Sit or stand with your back straight.
2. Imagine you're holding a large, heavy box in front of you.
3. Position your arms as if you're hugging this imaginary box.
4. Squeeze inward with your arms, engaging your chest and biceps.
5. Hold this position for 10-15 seconds.
6. Relax and repeat 3-5 times.

Troubleshooting Tip: If you have shoulder issues, keep the "box" lower, closer to your waist.

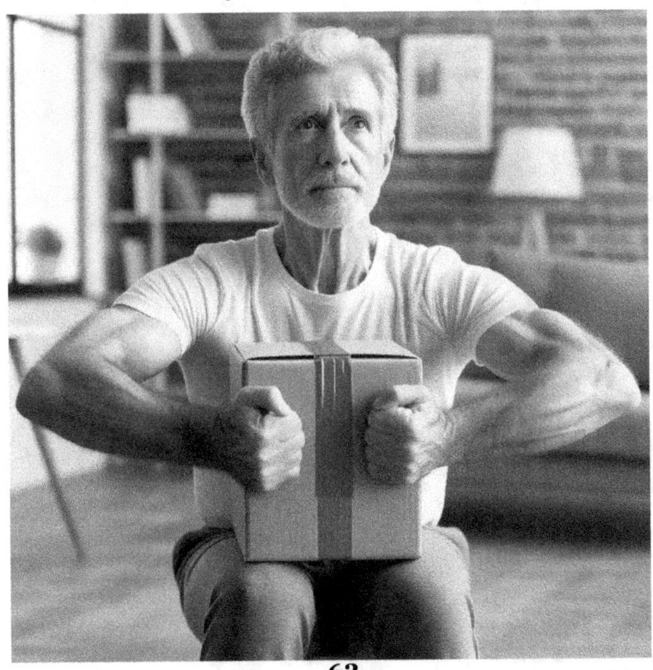

7. Wall Slide

This exercise combines arm and chest work with some shoulder mobility.

Steps:
1. Stand with your back against a wall, feet slightly away from the wall.
2. Raise your arms to shoulder height, bent at the elbows, so your upper arms are against the wall.
3. Slowly slide your arms up the wall as high as comfortable.
4. Hold at the top for 5-10 seconds, pressing your arms back against the wall.
5. Slowly slide back down to shoulder height.
6. Repeat 3-5 times.

Troubleshooting Tip: If you can't reach very high, that's okay. Work within your comfortable range of motion and try to increase it gradually over time.

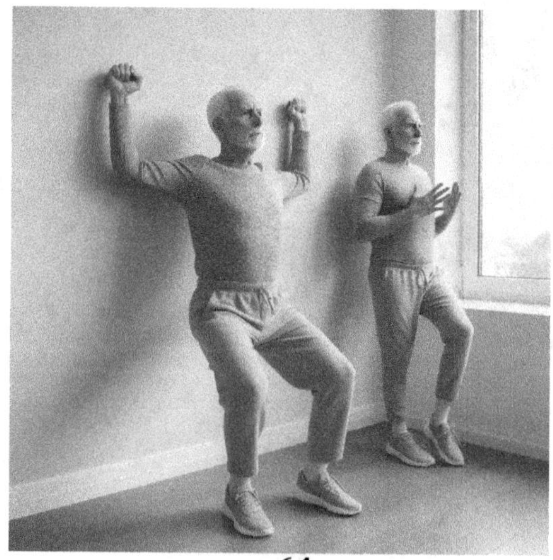

General Tips for Arm and Chest Exercises:

1. Warm-up: Start with gentle arm circles and shoulder rolls to prepare your muscles.
2. Maintain good posture: Keep your back straight and shoulders relaxed during exercises.
3. Breathe steadily: Don't hold your breath during the exercises.
4. Listen to your body: Stop if you feel any pain or excessive discomfort.
5. Consistency is key: Aim to do these exercises 2-3 times a week.
6. Progressive overload: Gradually increase hold times or resistance as you get stronger.

Troubleshooting Tip: If you have arthritis in your hands or wrists, try wearing compression gloves during exercises to provide extra support.

Remember, the goal is to build strength gradually and consistently. You're not competing with anyone but yourself. As you incorporate these exercises into your routine, you may notice improved arm strength, better chest muscle tone, and greater ease in daily activities that require upper body strength.

In our next section, we'll explore isometric exercises for the back and core. Are you feeling ready to give these arm and chest exercises a try? Wonderful! Let's continue our journey into the world of isometric exercise for seniors.

Imagine your back and core as the sturdy trunk of a tree, providing stability and support for your entire body. Strengthening these areas can improve posture, reduce back pain, and enhance overall balance. Let's dive into some effective isometric exercises for your back and core.

1. Wall Lean for Lower Back

This exercise targets your lower back muscles.

Steps:
1. Stand with your back against a wall, feet about 12 inches away from the wall.
2. Slide down the wall slightly, as if sitting in an invisible chair.
3. Press your lower back firmly against the wall.
4. Hold this position for 10-15 seconds, breathing normally.
5. Slowly slide back up.
6. Repeat 3-5 times.

Troubleshooting Tip: If this causes knee discomfort, try sliding down less. Even a small amount of lean can be effective.

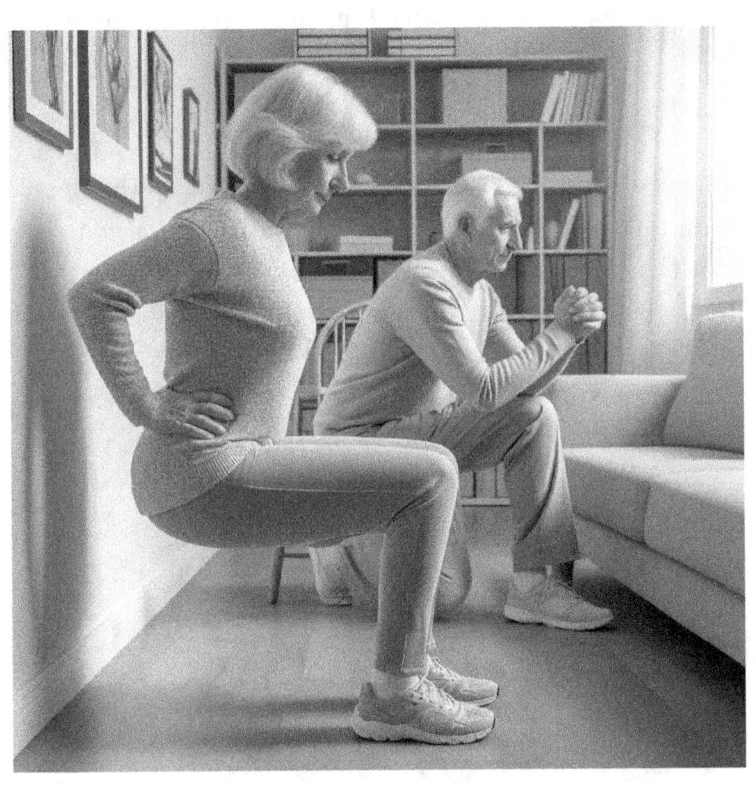

2. Seated Posture Hold

This exercise improves overall posture and engages your core.

Steps:
1. Sit on the edge of a chair with your feet flat on the floor.
2. Sit up tall, imagining a string pulling the top of your head towards the ceiling.
3. Pull your belly button towards your spine to engage your core.
4. Hold this posture for 15-20 seconds, breathing steadily.
5. Relax and repeat 3-5 times.

Troubleshooting Tip: If you feel strain in your neck, focus on lifting through your chest rather than your head.

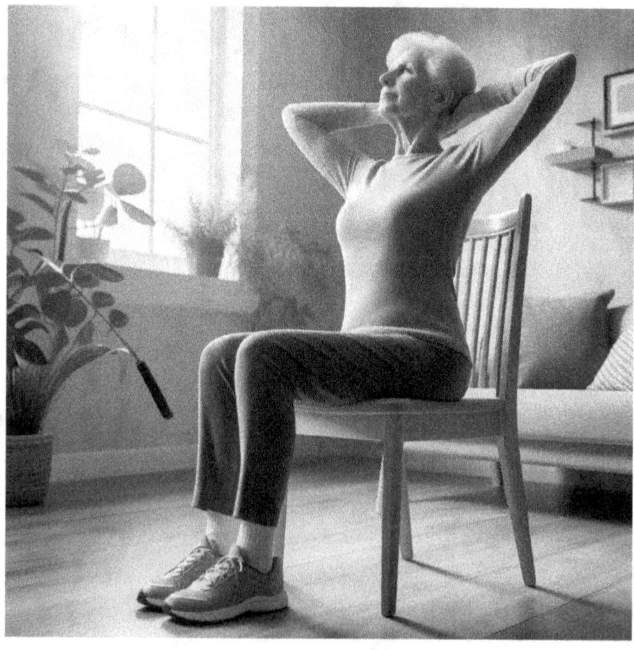

3. Tabletop Back Extension

This exercise strengthens your upper and middle back.

Steps:
1. Sit in a chair and lean forward, placing your hands on your thighs.
2. Keeping your lower back against the chair, try to arch your upper back.
3. Hold this position for 5-10 seconds.
4. Slowly return to the starting position.
5. Repeat 5-8 times.

Troubleshooting Tip: If you feel any neck strain, focus on moving from your upper back, not your neck.

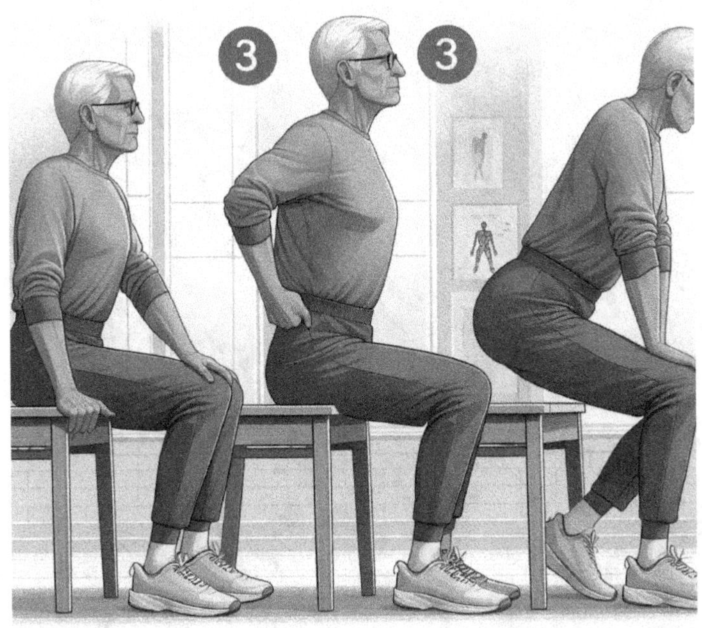

4. Stomach Vacuum

This exercise targets your deep core muscles.

Steps:
1. Sit comfortably in a chair with your back straight.
2. Exhale fully, drawing your belly button towards your spine.
3. Hold this "vacuum" position for 5-10 seconds while taking small breaths.
4. Relax and breathe normally for a few seconds.
5. Repeat 3-5 times.

Troubleshooting Tip: If you feel lightheaded, reduce the hold time and focus on taking slightly deeper breaths during the hold.

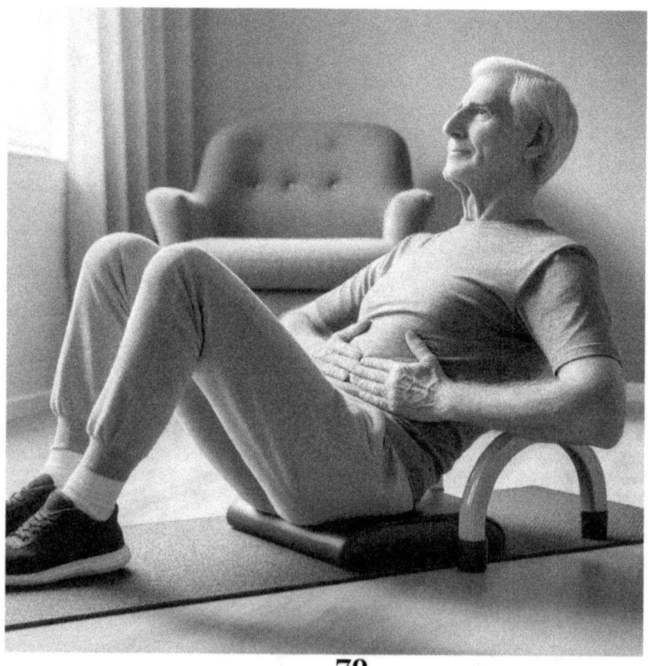

5. Seated Side Bend

This exercise works your obliques (side core muscles).

Steps:
1. Sit tall in a chair with your feet flat on the floor.
2. Place your right hand on the side of the chair seat.
3. Lift your left arm over your head, reaching to the right.
4. Hold this gentle side bend for 5-10 seconds.
5. Return to the starting position and repeat on the other side.
6. Do 3-5 repetitions on each side.

Troubleshooting Tip: If reaching overhead is uncomfortable, you can keep your arm lower and still get the benefits of the side bend.

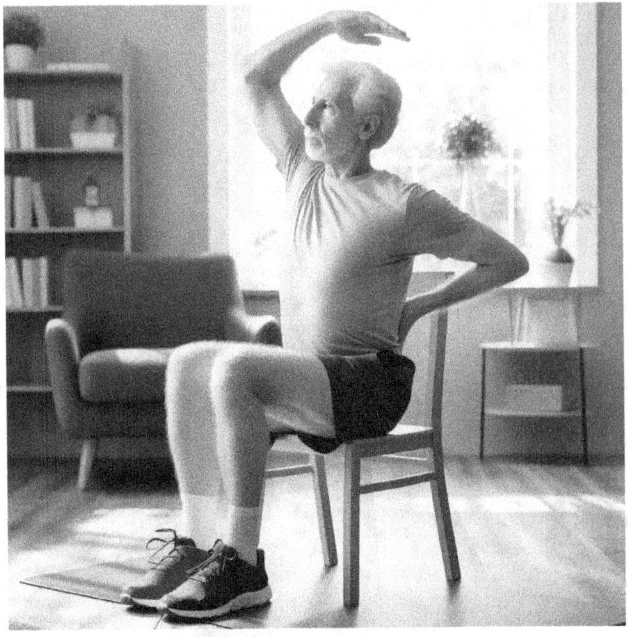

6. Chair Plank

This modified plank exercise engages your entire core.

Steps:
1. Stand facing the back of a sturdy chair.
2. Place your hands on the back of the chair, shoulder-width apart.
3. Step your feet back until your body forms a straight line from head to heels.
4. Engage your core by pulling your belly button towards your spine.
5. Hold this position for 10-15 seconds, breathing steadily.
6. Step forward to return to standing.
7. Repeat 3-5 times.

Troubleshooting Tip: If a full plank is too challenging, keep your knees on the ground for a modified version.

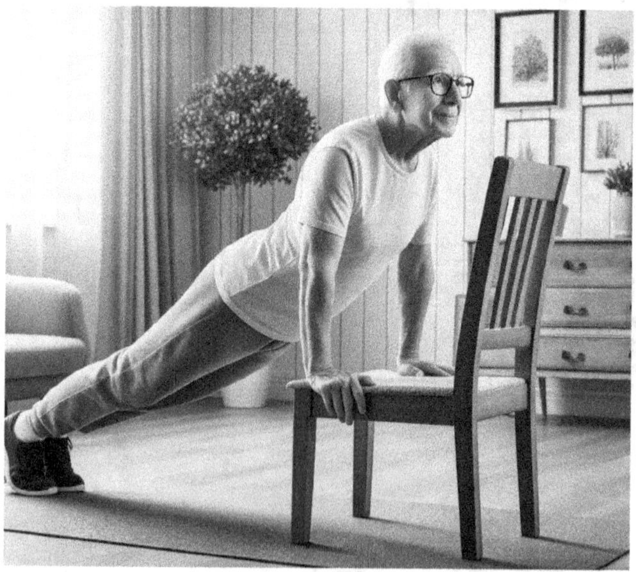

7. Seated Rotations

This exercise works your obliques and improves spinal mobility.

Steps:
1. Sit tall in a chair with your feet flat on the floor.
2. Cross your arms over your chest.
3. Slowly rotate your upper body to the right, keeping your hips facing forward.
4. Hold for 5 seconds.
5. Return to center, then rotate to the left.
6. Hold for 5 seconds.
7. Repeat 5-8 times on each side.

Troubleshooting Tip: If you experience any neck discomfort, try looking straight ahead instead of turning your head with your body.

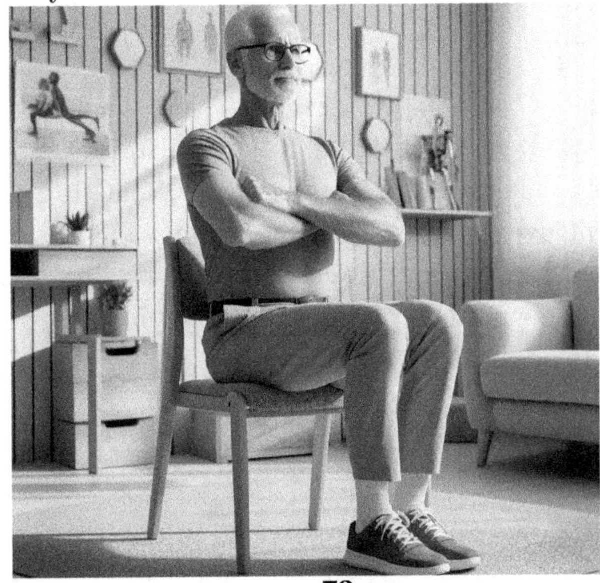

General Tips for Back and Core Exercises:

1. Warm-up: Start with gentle torso twists and shoulder rolls to prepare your muscles.
2. Maintain good posture: Keep your spine in a neutral position during exercises.
3. Breathe steadily: Focus on deep, steady breaths to support your core engagement.
4. Listen to your body: Stop if you feel any sharp pain, especially in your back.
5. Consistency is key: Aim to do these exercises 2-3 times a week.
6. Progressive overload: Gradually increase hold times as you get stronger.

Troubleshooting Tip: If you have chronic back pain, consult with a physical therapist or doctor before starting these exercises. They may need to be modified for your specific condition.

Remember, the goal of these exercises is to build strength and stability in your back and core gradually. You're not aiming for immediate, dramatic results, but for steady improvement over time. As you incorporate these exercises into your routine, you may notice improved posture, reduced back pain, and greater ease in daily activities that require core strength and stability.

Imagine your hips and glutes as the powerhouse of your lower body. These muscles play a crucial role in balance, mobility, and overall strength. Strengthening them can significantly improve your ability to walk, climb stairs, and perform daily activities with ease. Let's dive into some effective isometric exercises for your hips and glutes.

1. Wall Lean for Glutes

This exercise targets your gluteal muscles and helps improve hip stability.

Steps:
1. Stand with your back against a wall, feet about 12 inches from the wall.
2. Slide down the wall slightly, as if sitting in an invisible chair.
3. Squeeze your glutes (buttocks) together tightly.
4. Hold this position for 10-15 seconds, breathing normally.
5. Slowly slide back up the wall.
6. Repeat 3-5 times.

Troubleshooting Tip: If you feel strain in your knees, try sliding down the wall less. Even a small amount of lean can be effective.

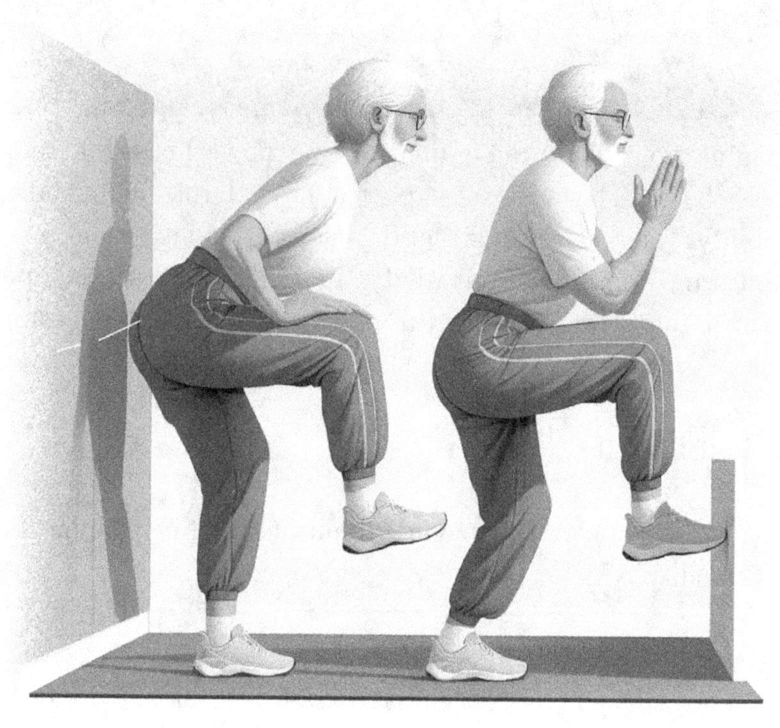

2. Standing Hip Abduction

This exercise strengthens the muscles on the outside of your hips, important for balance.

Steps:
1. Stand next to a wall or chair for support, feet hip-width apart.
2. Lift your right foot slightly off the ground.
3. Press the outside of your right foot against the wall or chair leg.
4. Hold this pressure for 10-15 seconds.
5. Relax and repeat on the left side.
6. Do 3-5 repetitions on each side.

Troubleshooting Tip: If you can't lift your foot, simply press the side of your foot against the wall or chair while keeping it on the ground.

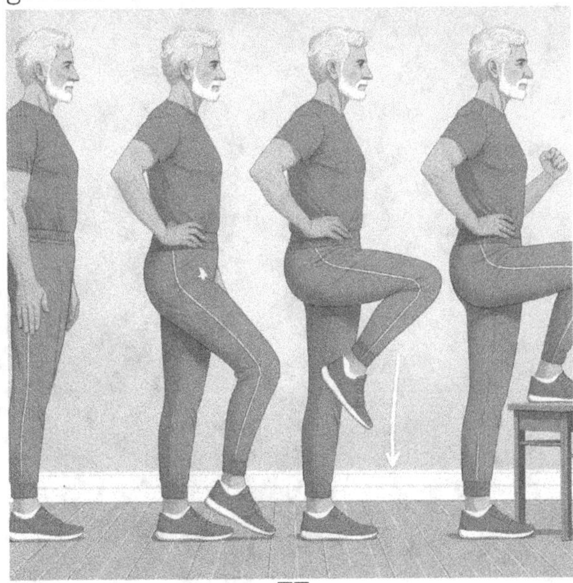

3. Seated Glute Squeeze

This simple exercise engages your glutes and can be done discreetly almost anywhere.

Steps:
1. Sit comfortably in a chair with your feet flat on the floor.
2. Squeeze your glutes (buttocks) together as tightly as you can.
3. Hold this contraction for 5-10 seconds.
4. Relax and repeat 8-10 times.

Troubleshooting Tip: If you have trouble feeling your glutes engage, try placing your hands under your buttocks to feel the muscles contract.

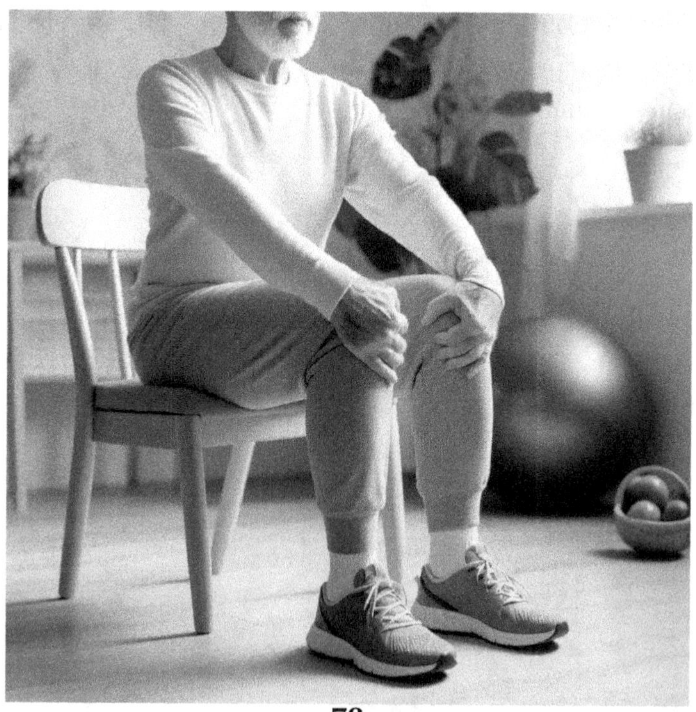

4. Hip Flexor Hold

This exercise targets the front of your hips, important for walking and climbing stairs.

Steps:
1. Sit on the edge of a chair with good posture.
2. Lift your right foot about 6 inches off the ground.
3. Hold this position for 10-15 seconds.
4. Lower your foot and repeat with the left leg.
5. Do 3-5 repetitions on each side.

Troubleshooting Tip: If lifting your foot is too challenging, try sliding your foot forward on the ground instead.

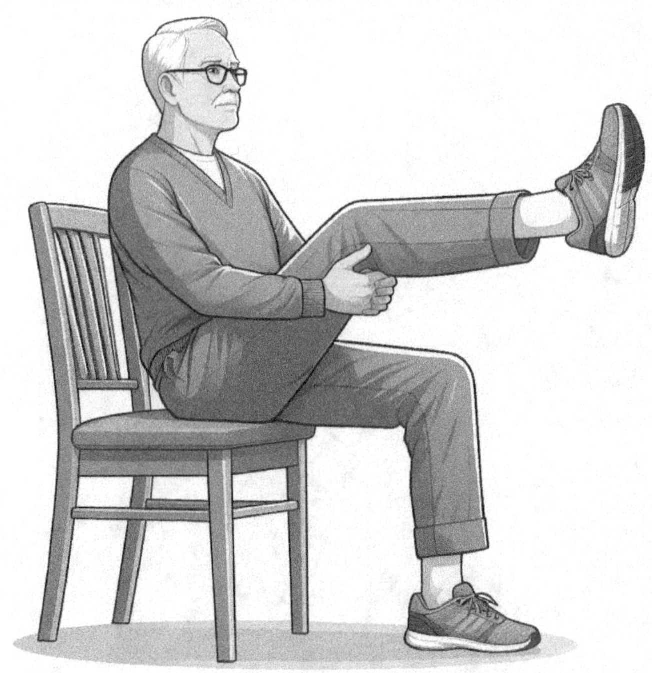

5. Bridge Hold

This exercise works your glutes, hamstrings, and core.

Steps:
1. Lie on your back with knees bent, feet flat on the floor.
2. Lift your hips off the ground until your body forms a straight line from knees to shoulders.
3. Squeeze your glutes tightly.
4. Hold this position for 10-15 seconds.
5. Slowly lower back down.
6. Repeat 3-5 times.

Troubleshooting Tip: If a full bridge is too challenging, try lifting your hips just a few inches off the ground.

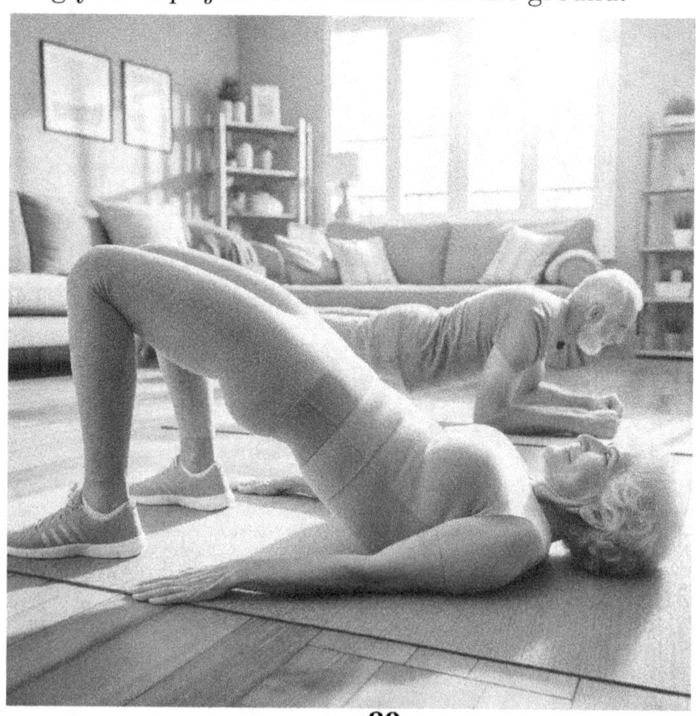

6. Standing Hip Extension

This exercise targets your glutes and the back of your hips.

Steps:
1. Stand facing a wall or chair, holding on for balance.
2. Shift your weight onto your left leg.
3. Lift your right foot slightly off the ground and move it back a few inches.
4. Press your right heel back, as if trying to make a footprint on a wall behind you.
5. Hold this position for 10-15 seconds.
6. Return to the starting position and repeat on the other side.
7. Do 3-5 repetitions on each side.

Troubleshooting Tip: Keep your back straight and avoid leaning forward. The movement should come from your hip, not your lower back.

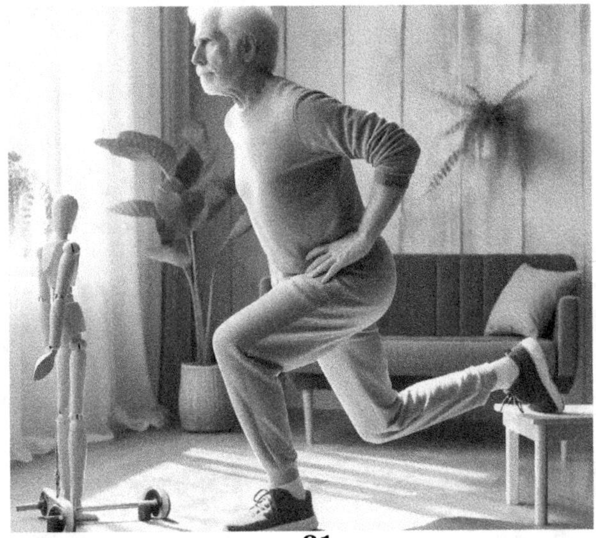

7. Seated Marching

This exercise engages your hip flexors and core muscles.

Steps:
1. Sit tall in a chair with your feet flat on the floor.
2. Lift your right knee up towards your chest, holding it there with your hands.
3. Push your knee into your hands while resisting with your arms.
4. Hold for 5-10 seconds.
5. Lower your right foot and repeat with the left leg.
6. Alternate legs, doing 5-8 repetitions on each side.

Troubleshooting Tip: If you can't lift your knee high, even a small lift will provide benefits. Work within your comfortable range of motion.

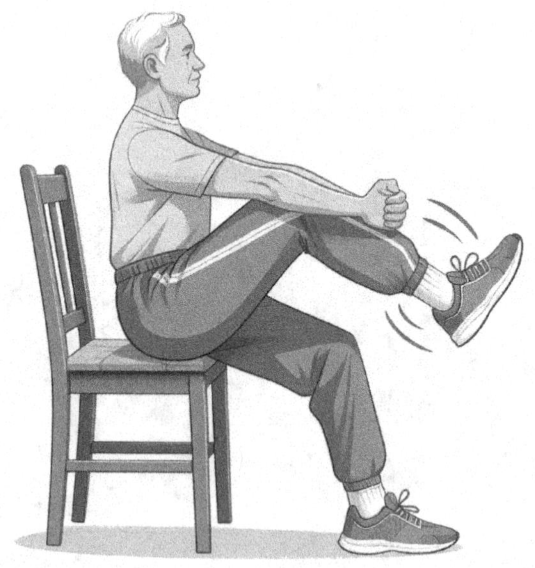

General Tips for Hip and Glute Exercises:
1. Warm-up: Start with gentle hip circles and leg swings to prepare your muscles.
2. Maintain good posture: Keep your spine neutral and engage your core during exercises.
3. Breathe steadily: Focus on deep, steady breaths to support your effort.
4. Listen to your body: Stop if you feel any sharp pain, especially in your hips or lower back.
5. Consistency is key: Aim to do these exercises 2-3 times a week.
6. Progressive overload: Gradually increase hold times as you get stronger.

Troubleshooting Tip: If you have hip arthritis or have had a hip replacement, consult with your doctor or physical therapist before starting these exercises. They may need to be modified for your specific condition.

Remember, the goal of these exercises is to build strength and stability in your hips and glutes gradually. You're not aiming for immediate, dramatic results, but for steady improvement over time. As you incorporate these exercises into your routine, you may notice improved balance, easier walking, and greater ease in activities like standing up from a chair or climbing stairs.

In our next section, we'll explore isometric exercises for the thighs and knees. Are you feeling ready to give these hip and glute exercises a try? Wonderful! Let's continue our journey into the world of isometric exercise for seniors.

Imagine your thighs and knees as the sturdy pillars supporting your body. Strengthening these areas can significantly improve your ability to walk, climb stairs, and maintain balance. Let's dive into some effective isometric exercises for your thighs and knees.

1. Wall Sit

This classic exercise targets your quadriceps (front thigh muscles) and helps strengthen the knees.

Steps:
1. Stand with your back against a wall, feet shoulder-width apart and about 2 feet from the wall.
2. Slowly slide your back down the wall until your thighs are parallel to the ground, as if sitting in an invisible chair.
3. Ensure your knees are directly above your ankles, not extending past your toes.
4. Hold this position for 10-30 seconds, depending on your strength.
5. Slowly slide back up to the starting position.
6. Repeat 3-5 times.

Troubleshooting Tip: If a full wall sit is too challenging, don't slide down as far. Even a slight bend in the knees will provide benefits.

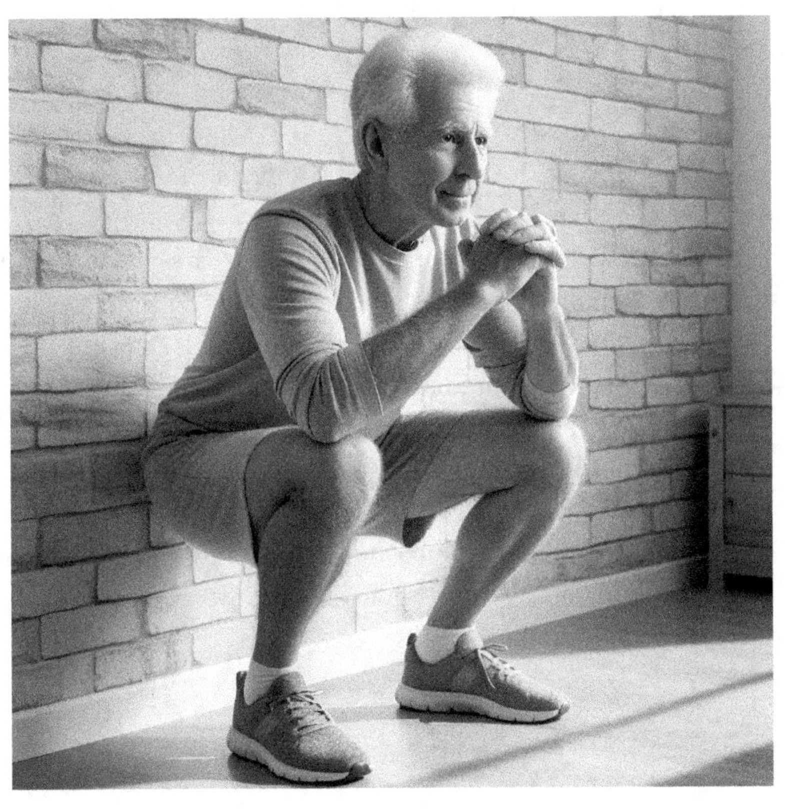

2. Seated Leg Extension

This exercise strengthens your quadriceps and the muscles around your knees.

Steps:
1. Sit in a chair with your back straight and feet flat on the floor.
2. Slowly lift your right foot until your leg is straight (or as straight as comfortable).
3. Tighten your thigh muscles and hold for 5-10 seconds.
4. Slowly lower your foot back to the starting position.
5. Repeat with your left leg.
6. Do 5-8 repetitions with each leg.

Troubleshooting Tip: If you can't fully straighten your leg, lift it as high as comfortable. The key is to feel the contraction in your thigh.

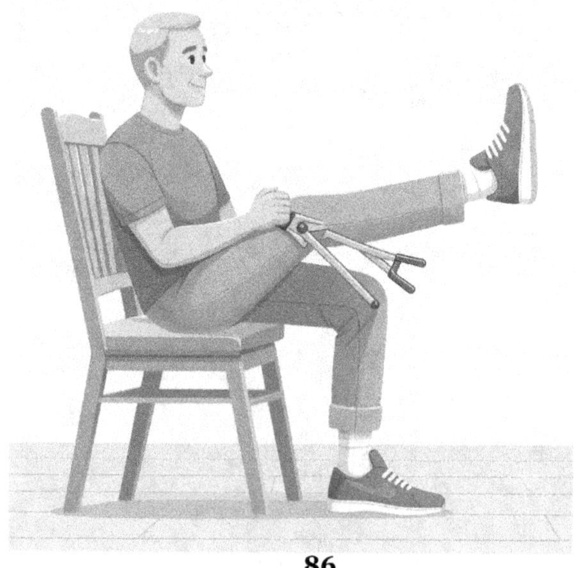

3. Inner Thigh Squeeze

This exercise targets your adductor muscles (inner thighs).

Steps:
1. Sit in a chair with your back straight.
2. Place a small pillow or rolled towel between your knees.
3. Squeeze your knees together, compressing the pillow.
4. Hold this contraction for 5-10 seconds.
5. Relax and repeat 8-10 times.

Troubleshooting Tip: If you don't have a pillow, you can perform this exercise without one, simply squeezing your knees together.

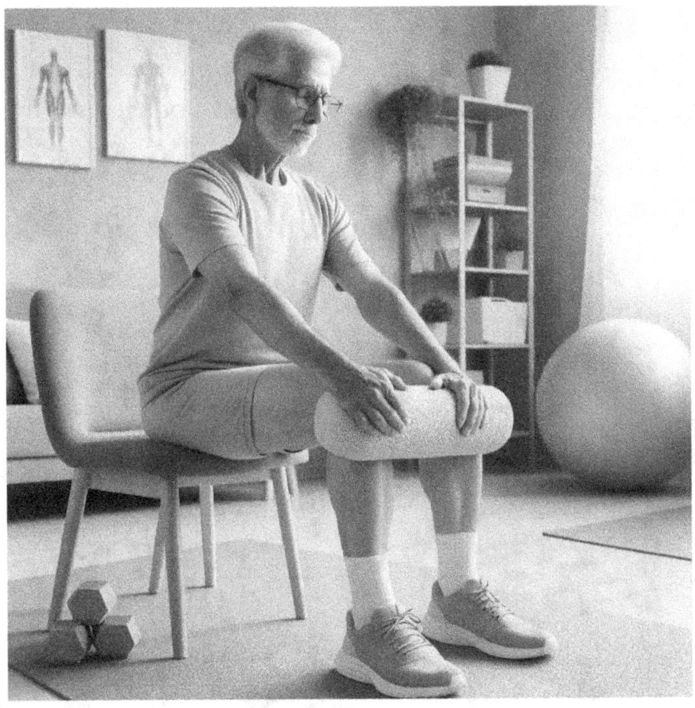

4. Standing Hamstring Curl

This exercise works your hamstrings (back of thigh) and helps with knee stability.

Steps:
1. Stand behind a chair, holding onto it for balance.
2. Shift your weight onto your left leg.
3. Bend your right knee, bringing your heel towards your buttocks.
4. Hold this position for 5-10 seconds.
5. Slowly lower your foot back to the ground.
6. Repeat with your left leg.
7. Do 5-8 repetitions with each leg.

Troubleshooting Tip: If you can't lift your heel very high, even a small bend in the knee will engage your hamstrings.

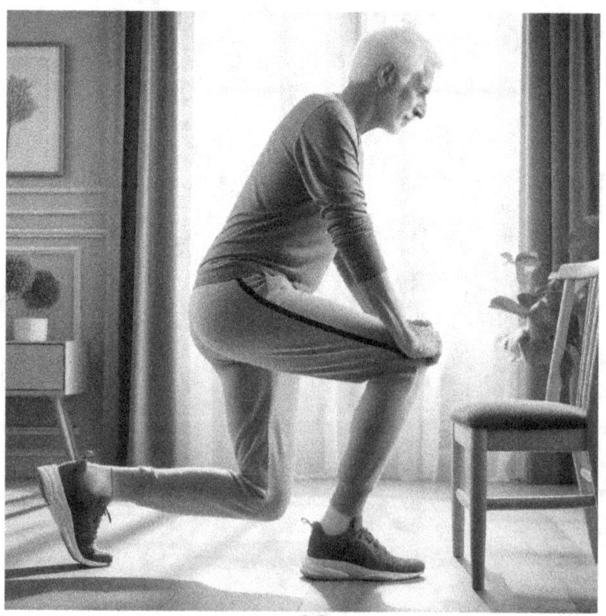

5. Isometric Squat Hold

This exercise engages multiple leg muscles and helps improve overall lower body strength.

Steps:
1. Stand with feet shoulder-width apart.
2. Slowly lower your body as if you're about to sit in a chair, lowering until your thighs are parallel to the ground (or as low as comfortable).
3. Hold this position for 10-30 seconds.
4. Slowly return to the starting position.
5. Repeat 3-5 times.

Troubleshooting Tip: If a full squat is too challenging, try a partial squat. Even a slight bend in the knees will provide benefits.

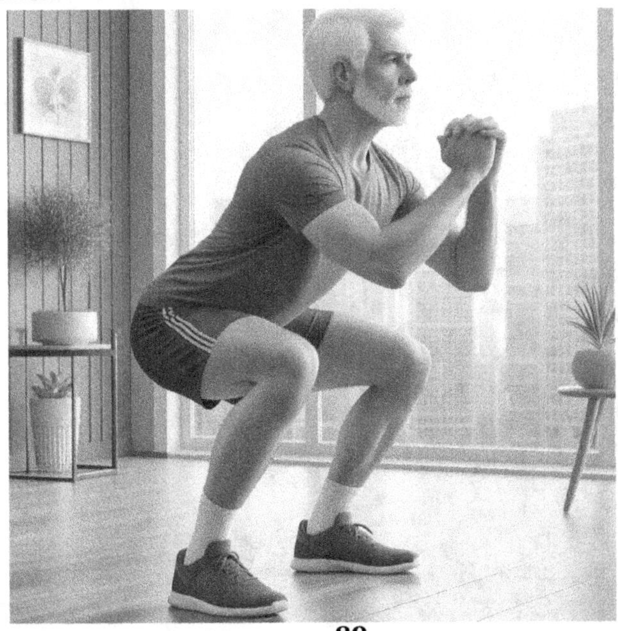

6. Seated Knee Press

This exercise helps strengthen the muscles around your knees.

Steps:
1. Sit in a chair with your back straight and feet flat on the floor.
2. Place a rolled towel or small pillow under your right knee.
3. Press your knee down into the towel, engaging your thigh muscles.
4. Hold for 5-10 seconds.
5. Relax and repeat with your left leg.
6. Do 5-8 repetitions with each leg.

Troubleshooting Tip: If you feel any pain in your knee, reduce the pressure or try placing the towel behind your knee instead of under it.

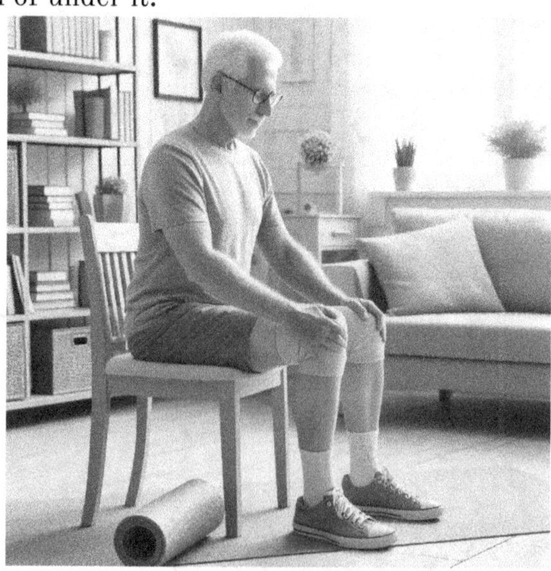

7. Wall Calf Raise Hold

While primarily a calf exercise, this also engages your thighs
and improves knee stability.

Steps:
1. Stand facing a wall, about arm's length away.
2. Place your hands on the wall for balance.
3. Slowly rise up onto your toes.
4. Hold this position for 10-15 seconds.
5. Slowly lower back down.
6. Repeat 5-8 times.

Troubleshooting Tip: If balance is a concern, you can do this
exercise while holding onto a sturdy chair instead of a wall.

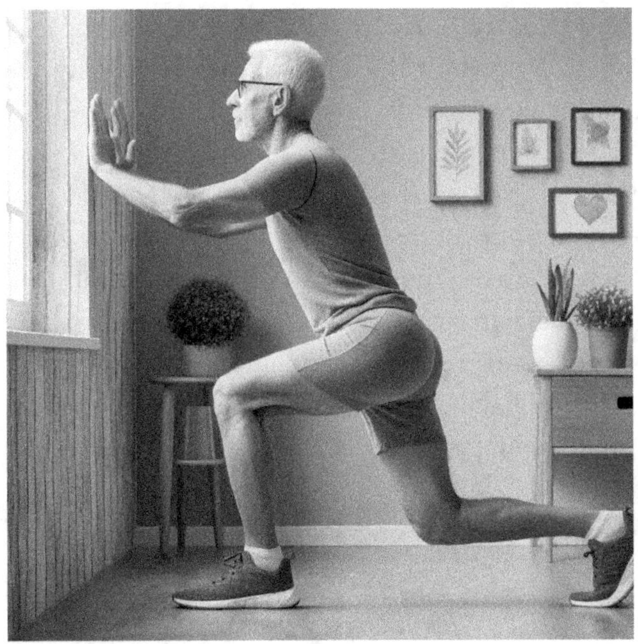

General Tips for Thigh and Knee Exercises:

1. Warm-up: Start with gentle leg swings and knee circles to prepare your muscles.
2. Maintain good posture: Keep your back straight and engage your core during exercises.
3. Breathe steadily: Avoid holding your breath during the exercises.
4. Listen to your body: Stop if you feel any sharp pain, especially in your knees.
5. Consistency is key: Aim to do these exercises 2-3 times a week.
6. Progressive overload: Gradually increase hold times as you get stronger.

Troubleshooting Tip: If you have arthritis or have had knee replacement surgery, consult with your doctor or physical therapist before starting these exercises. They may need to be modified for your specific condition.

Remember, the goal of these exercises is to build strength and stability in your thighs and around your knees gradually. You're not aiming for immediate, dramatic results, but for steady improvement over time. As you incorporate these exercises into your routine, you may notice improved leg strength, better balance, and greater ease in activities like walking and climbing stairs.

Imagine your calves and ankles as the foundation of your body's mobility. Strong, flexible calves and ankles can significantly improve your balance, walking ability, and overall lower body strength. Let's dive into some effective isometric exercises for your calves and ankles.

1. Standing Calf Raise Hold

This exercise strengthens your calf muscles and improves ankle stability.

Steps:
1. Stand behind a chair, holding onto it for balance.
2. Slowly rise up onto your toes, lifting your heels off the ground.
3. Hold this position for 10-15 seconds.
4. Slowly lower your heels back to the ground.
5. Repeat 5-8 times.

Troubleshooting Tip: If you can't lift your heels very high, even a small lift will engage your calf muscles. Focus on stability rather than height.

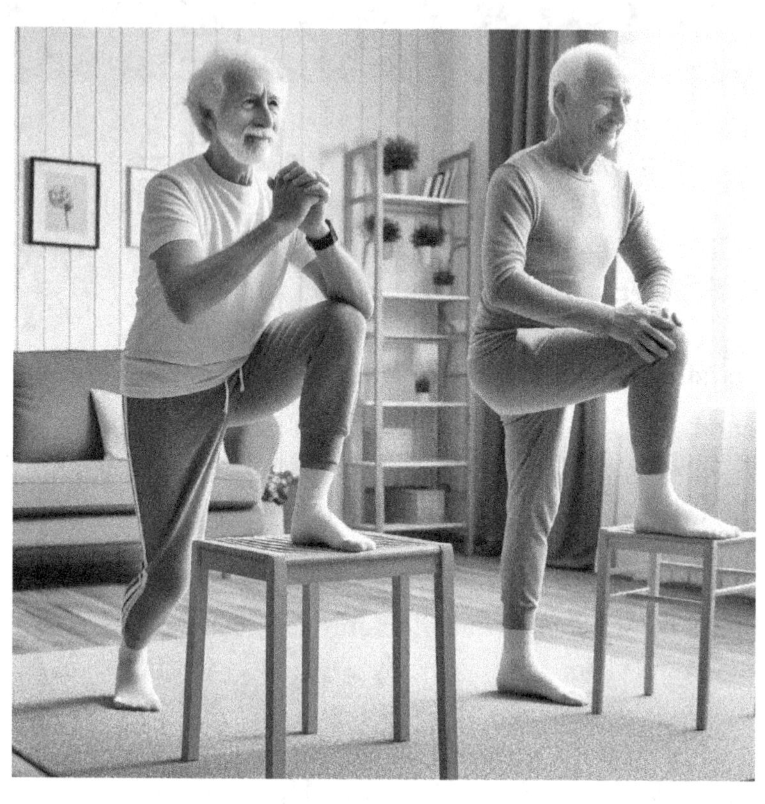

2. Seated Ankle Rotations

This exercise improves ankle flexibility and strength.

Steps:
1. Sit comfortably in a chair with your feet flat on the floor.
2. Lift your right foot slightly off the ground.
3. Rotate your ankle in a circular motion clockwise 5 times.
4. Hold your ankle in the fully flexed position (toes pointing up) for 5-10 seconds.
5. Rotate your ankle counterclockwise 5 times.
6. Hold your ankle in the fully extended position (toes pointing down) for 5-10 seconds.
7. Repeat with your left foot.

Troubleshooting Tip: If you experience any cramping, gently massage your calf and take a short break before continuing.

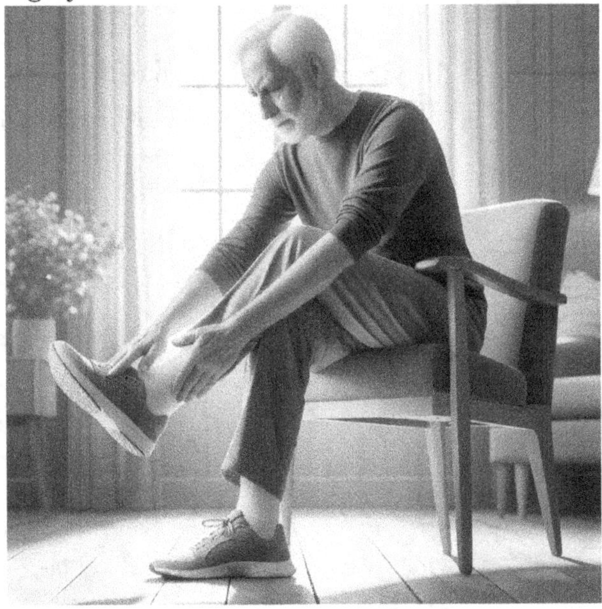

3. Wall Calf Stretch with Isometric Hold

This exercise combines stretching and strengthening for your calves.

Steps:
1. Stand facing a wall, about arm's length away.
2. Step your right foot back, keeping it straight, while bending your left knee slightly.
3. Lean forward, placing your hands on the wall.
4. Keep your back heel on the ground to feel a stretch in your right calf.
5. While in this position, try to push your back heel into the ground.
6. Hold this isometric contraction for 10-15 seconds.
7. Relax and repeat with the left leg.
8. Do 3-5 repetitions on each side.

Troubleshooting Tip: If you can't keep your heel on the ground, it's okay to lift it slightly. The key is to feel a gentle stretch in your calf.

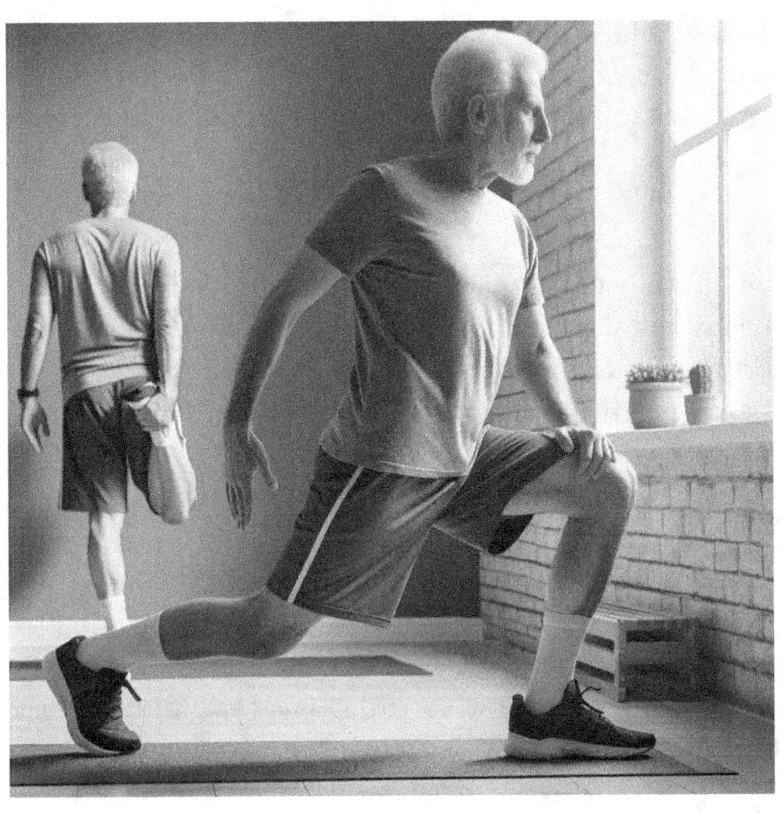

4. Towel Ankle Pull

This exercise strengthens the muscles at the front of your lower leg.

Steps:
1. Sit on the floor with your legs straight out in front of you.
2. Loop a towel around the ball of your right foot.
3. Hold the ends of the towel with both hands.
4. Gently pull the towel towards you while pushing your foot against the resistance.
5. Hold this isometric contraction for 5-10 seconds.
6. Relax and repeat 5-8 times.
7. Switch to the left foot and repeat.

Troubleshooting Tip: If sitting on the floor is uncomfortable, you can do this exercise while sitting in a chair with your leg extended.

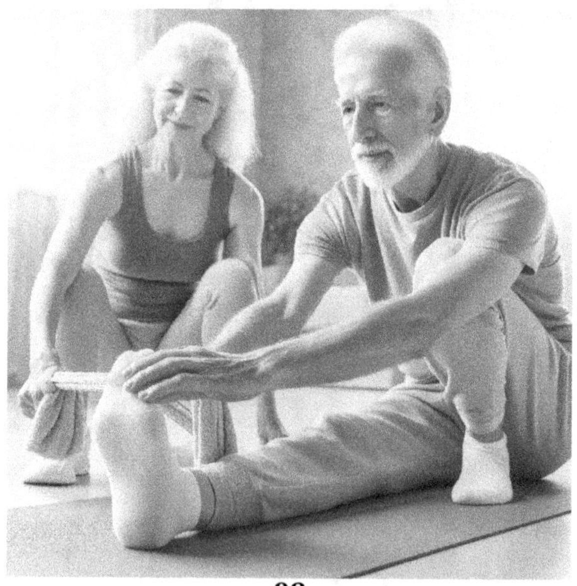

5. Seated Calf Press

This exercise targets your calf muscles in a seated position.

Steps:
1. Sit in a chair with your feet flat on the floor.
2. Lift your heels off the ground, keeping the balls of your feet on the floor.
3. Press your toes firmly into the ground.
4. Hold this position for 10-15 seconds.
5. Slowly lower your heels.
6. Repeat 5-8 times.

Troubleshooting Tip: If you can't lift both heels at once, try alternating: lift one heel at a time.

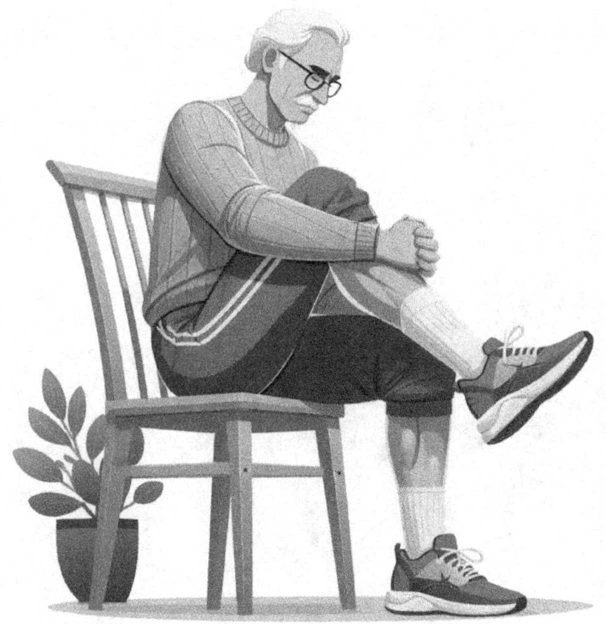

6. Ankle Alphabet

This exercise improves ankle mobility and strength.

Steps:
1. Sit comfortably in a chair with your feet slightly off the ground.
2. Using your right foot, "write" the alphabet in the air with your big toe.
3. Try to move only your ankle, keeping your leg still.
4. After completing the alphabet, hold your ankle in a flexed position (toes pointing up) for 5-10 seconds.
5. Repeat with your left foot.

Troubleshooting Tip: If doing the full alphabet is too tiring, start with just a few letters and gradually work up to more.

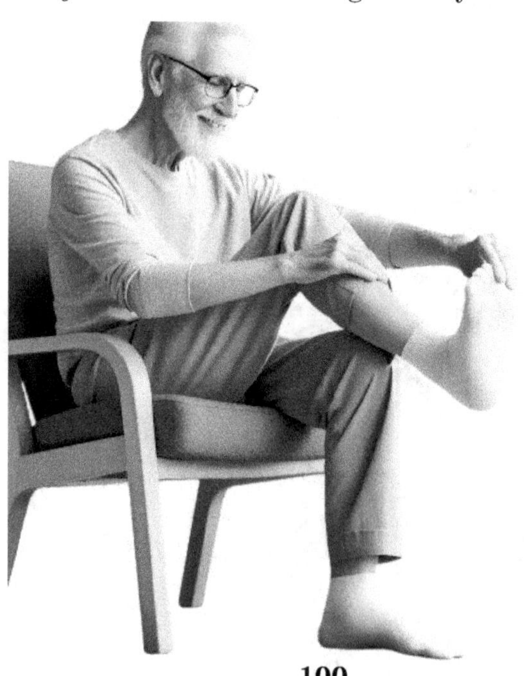

7. Standing Ankle Dorsiflexion

This exercise strengthens the muscles at the front of your lower leg.

Steps:
1. Stand with your back against a wall for support.
2. Keeping your right heel on the ground, lift the front of your right foot as high as you can.
3. Hold this position for 5-10 seconds.
4. Slowly lower your foot.
5. Repeat 5-8 times, then switch to the left foot.

Troubleshooting Tip: If you can't lift your foot very high, that's okay. Even a small lift will engage the targeted muscles.

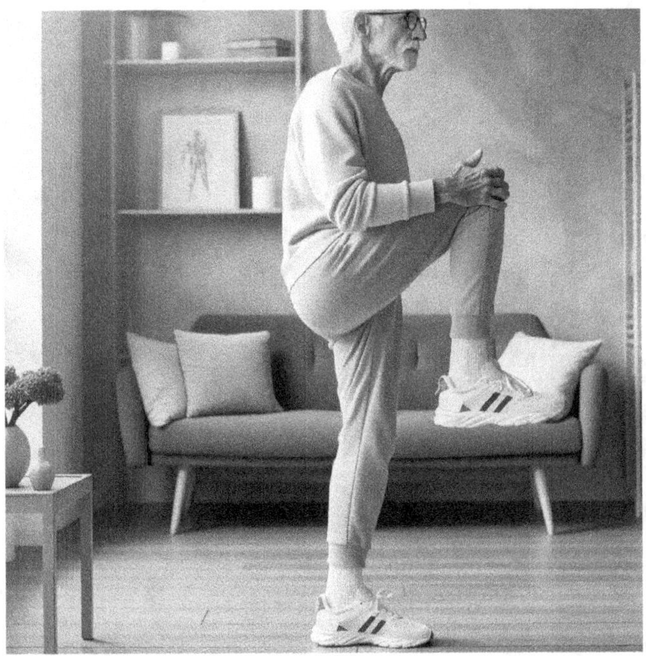

General Tips for Calf and Ankle Exercises:

1. Warm-up: Start with gentle ankle rotations and calf stretches to prepare your muscles.
2. Maintain good posture: Keep your back straight and engage your core during standing exercises.
3. Breathe steadily: Remember to breathe normally throughout the exercises.
4. Listen to your body: Stop if you feel any sharp pain or excessive discomfort.
5. Consistency is key: Aim to do these exercises 2-3 times a week.
6. Progressive overload: Gradually increase hold times and repetitions as you get stronger.

Troubleshooting Tip: If you have any foot conditions (like plantar fasciitis) or have had recent ankle injuries, consult with your doctor or a physical therapist before starting these exercises.

Remember, the goal of these exercises is to build strength and flexibility in your calves and ankles gradually. You're not aiming for immediate, dramatic results, but for steady improvement over time. As you incorporate these exercises into your routine, you may notice improved balance, easier walking, and reduced risk of falls.

Chapter 5
Full-Body Isometric Routines

10-minute morning energizer

Imagine starting your day with a gentle yet effective workout that leaves you feeling invigorated and ready to tackle whatever lies ahead. This 10-minute routine does just that, engaging all major muscle groups without the need for any equipment.

Preparation:
- Wear comfortable clothing
- Have a chair nearby for balance if needed
- Keep a glass of water handy

Warm-Up (1 minute):
Begin with gentle movements to wake up your body:
1. March in place for 30 seconds, lifting your knees as high as comfortable
2. Roll your shoulders backward 5 times, then forward 5 times
3. Gently twist your torso side to side 5 times

Now, let's move into the main routine. Perform each exercise for 30 seconds, followed by 10 seconds of rest before moving to the next exercise.

1. Wall Push (Upper Body) - 30 seconds

Steps:
1. Stand arm's length from a wall
2. Place your palms flat against the wall at shoulder height
3. Lean in slightly and push against the wall
4. Hold this position, breathing steadily

Troubleshooting Tip: If your wrists feel strained, make a fist and push with your knuckles instead.

2. Chair Squat Hold (Lower Body) - 30 seconds

Steps:
1. Stand in front of a chair as if you're about to sit
2. Lower yourself until you're barely touching the chair
3. Hold this position, keeping your weight in your heels
4. Keep your chest up and core engaged

Troubleshooting Tip: If this is too challenging, rest lightly on the chair while maintaining the squat position.

3. Plank on Wall (Core) - 30 seconds

Steps:
1. Stand facing a wall and place your forearms against it
2. Walk your feet back until your body forms a straight line
3. Push your forearms into the wall and engage your core
4. Hold this position, breathing steadily

Troubleshooting Tip: The further you walk your feet back, the more challenging this becomes. Find a comfortable angle for you.

4. Doorway Chest Stretch (Upper Body) - 30 seconds

Steps:
1. Stand in an open doorway
2. Raise your arms to the sides at shoulder height
3. Place your palms on the door frame
4. Lean forward slightly until you feel a stretch in your chest
5. Hold this position, breathing deeply

Troubleshooting Tip: If you can't reach the top of the doorway, lower your arms to a comfortable height.

5. Calf Raise Hold (Lower Body) - 30 seconds

Steps:
1. Stand behind a chair, holding it lightly for balance
2. Rise up onto your toes
3. Hold this position, keeping your core engaged
4. Focus on balance and stability

Troubleshooting Tip: If you can't rise fully onto your toes, even a small lift will engage your calf muscles.

6. Seated Spinal Twist (Core/Back) - 30 seconds

Steps:
1. Sit sideways in a chair with your feet flat on the floor
2. Twist your torso to face the back of the chair
3. Hold the back of the chair gently for support
4. Hold this twist, breathing deeply
5. Switch sides after 15 seconds

Troubleshooting Tip: Only twist as far as is comfortable. The goal is a gentle stretch, not maximum rotation.

7. Wall Sit (Lower Body) - 30 seconds

Steps:
1. Lean your back against a wall
2. Slide down until your thighs are parallel to the ground
3. Ensure your knees are above your ankles
4. Hold this position, keeping your core engaged

Troubleshooting Tip: If a full wall sit is too challenging, don't slide down as far. Even a slight bend in the knees will be beneficial.

8. Overhead Press on Wall (Upper Body) - 30 seconds

Steps:
1. Stand facing a wall, about arm's length away
2. Place your palms on the wall at shoulder height
3. Press upward against the wall
4. Hold this position, engaging your shoulder and arm muscles

Troubleshooting Tip: If reaching overhead is uncomfortable, lower your hands to a position that feels comfortable.

9. Standing Core Engagement (Core) - 30 seconds

Steps:
1. Stand with your feet hip-width apart
2. Place your hands on your hips
3. Imagine pulling your belly button toward your spine
4. Hold this engagement, breathing steadily

Troubleshooting Tip: If you're unsure about engaging your core, imagine preparing for someone to punch your stomach (gently!).

10. Full Body Stretch - 30 seconds

Steps:
1. Stand tall with feet hip-width apart
2. Raise your arms overhead, interlacing your fingers
3. Push your palms toward the ceiling
4. Rise onto your toes if balance allows
5. Hold this full-body stretch, breathing deeply

Troubleshooting Tip: If balance is a concern, keep your feet flat on the ground and focus on the upper body stretch.

Cool Down (1 minute):
- March in place gently for 30 seconds
- Take 3 deep breaths, inhaling through your nose and exhaling through your mouth

Remember to drink water after completing your routine. This 10-minute energizer is designed to wake up your body and mind, preparing you for the day ahead. As you become more comfortable with the routine, you can increase the hold times or add more challenging variations of each exercise.

Consistency is key – try to perform this routine every morning, and you'll likely notice improvements in your energy levels, strength, and overall well-being over time. Are you ready to energize your mornings with this isometric routine? Let's make it a healthy habit!

Imagine feeling more confident and steady on your feet, able to navigate your daily activities with greater ease and reduced fear of falling. This 15-minute routine is designed to improve your balance, enhance proprioception (your body's sense of position), and strengthen the muscles that support stability.

Preparation:
- Wear comfortable, non-slip shoes
- Have a sturdy chair nearby for support
- Keep a glass of water handy
- Clear the area of any tripping hazards

Warm-Up (2 minutes):
1. March in place for 30 seconds, focusing on lifting your knees
2. Ankle rotations: 5 circles in each direction with each foot
3. Shoulder rolls: 5 backward, 5 forward
4. Gentle side-to-side neck tilts: 5 on each side

Now, let's move into the main routine. Perform each exercise for 45 seconds, followed by 15 seconds of rest before moving to the next exercise.

1. Single Leg Stand (Right) - 45 seconds

Steps:
1. Stand behind a chair, holding it lightly for support
2. Slowly lift your right foot off the ground

3. Hold this position, focusing on keeping your standing leg straight and your posture upright
4. If stable, try releasing your hand from the chair

Troubleshooting Tip: If lifting your foot is too challenging, start by just shifting your weight onto one leg while keeping both feet on the ground.

2. Single Leg Stand (Left) - 45 seconds

Repeat the same exercise on the left side.

3. Heel-to-Toe Stand - 45 seconds

Steps:
1. Stand with the heel of your right foot touching the toes of your left foot
2. Place your arms out to the sides for balance
3. Hold this position, focusing on staying steady
4. If stable, try closing your eyes for a few seconds at a time

Troubleshooting Tip: If touching heel to toe is too difficult, start with your feet closer together but not touching.

4. Wall Lean with Head Turns - 45 seconds

Steps:
1. Stand with your back against a wall, feet about 6 inches away from the wall
2. Slowly turn your head to look over your right shoulder
3. Hold for 5 seconds, then turn to look over your left shoulder

4. Continue alternating sides

Troubleshooting Tip: If you feel dizzy, make smaller head movements or keep your eyes fixed on a point in front of you.

5. Toe Taps - 45 seconds

Steps:
1. Stand behind a chair, holding it for support
2. Slowly tap your right toe out to the side, then return it to the center
3. Repeat with your left toe
4. Continue alternating sides

Troubleshooting Tip: Focus on keeping your core engaged and your standing leg steady as you move your foot.

6. Flamingo Stand (Right) - 45 seconds

Steps:
1. Stand on your right leg, holding a chair for support
2. Bend your left knee, bringing your foot behind you
3. Hold this position, focusing on keeping your standing leg straight
4. If stable, try releasing your hand from the chair

Troubleshooting Tip: If you can't lift your foot behind you, simply shift your weight onto your right leg while keeping both feet on the ground.

7. Flamingo Stand (Left) - 45 seconds

Repeat the same exercise on the left side.

8. Clock Reach - 45 seconds

Steps:
1. Imagine you're standing in the center of a clock
2. Keeping both feet on the ground, reach your right hand towards 12 o'clock
3. Return to center, then reach towards 3 o'clock
4. Continue reaching to different "hours" on the clock

Troubleshooting Tip: Make your reaches smaller if you feel unsteady, and use a chair for support if needed.

9. Heel-Toe Walk - 45 seconds

Steps:
1. Stand at one end of a room, with a wall or furniture nearby for support if needed
2. Walk forward, placing the heel of one foot directly in front of the toes of your other foot
3. Take 5-10 steps forward, then walk backward to your starting position

Troubleshooting Tip: If this is too challenging, start by just practicing the heel-toe stance without walking.

10. Standing Weight Shifts - 45 seconds

Steps:
1. Stand with your feet hip-width apart
2. Slowly shift your weight to your right foot, lifting your left foot slightly
3. Hold for 5 seconds, then shift your weight to your left foot
4. Continue alternating sides

Troubleshooting Tip: Keep your movements slow and controlled, and use a chair for support if needed.

Cool Down (2 minutes):
1. March in place gently for 30 seconds
2. Ankle rolls: 5 in each direction for each foot
3. Shoulder shrugs: 5 repetitions
4. Deep breathing: Take 3 deep breaths, inhaling through your nose and exhaling through your mouth

Remember to drink water after completing your routine. This 15-minute balance improver is designed to challenge your stability in a safe, controlled manner. As you become more comfortable with the routine, you can increase the difficulty by:

- Holding positions for longer
- Reducing your reliance on the chair for support
- Closing your eyes during static balance exercises (only if you feel safe doing so)

Consistency is key – try to perform this routine 2-3 times a week, and you'll likely notice improvements in your balance, coordination, and overall confidence in movement. Always prioritize safety and listen to your body. If you ever feel excessively dizzy or unsteady, stop the exercise and consult with your healthcare provider.

Are you ready to improve your balance with this isometric routine? Let's make steady progress towards better stability and confidence in your daily activities!

Imagine feeling stronger and more capable in your everyday life, able to perform daily tasks with greater ease and confidence. This 20-minute routine is designed to build strength throughout your body using safe, effective isometric exercises.

Preparation:
- Wear comfortable clothing and supportive shoes
- Have a sturdy chair and a wall space nearby
- Keep a glass of water handy
- Have a towel or small pillow available

Warm-Up (3 minutes):
1. March in place for 45 seconds, gradually increasing knee lift
2. Arm circles: 10 forward, 10 backward
3. Gentle torso twists: 10 to each side
4. Shoulder shrugs: 10 repetitions
5. Ankle rotations: 5 circles in each direction with each foot

Now, let's move into the main routine. Perform each exercise for 45 seconds, followed by 15 seconds of rest before moving to the next exercise.

1. Wall Push (Upper Body) - 45 seconds

Steps:
1. Stand arm's length from a wall
2. Place your palms flat against the wall at shoulder height
3. Lean in slightly and push against the wall
4. Hold this position, engaging your chest and arm muscles

Troubleshooting Tip: If your wrists feel strained, make fists and push with your knuckles instead.

2. Chair Squat Hold (Lower Body) - 45 seconds

Steps:
1. Stand in front of a chair
2. Lower yourself as if about to sit, stopping just before you touch the chair
3. Hold this position, keeping your weight in your heels
4. Keep your chest up and core engaged

Troubleshooting Tip: If holding the squat is too challenging, rest lightly on the chair while maintaining the squat position.

3. Plank on Wall (Core) - 45 seconds

Steps:
1. Stand facing a wall and place your forearms against it
2. Walk your feet back until your body forms a straight line
3. Push your forearms into the wall and engage your core
4. Hold this position, keeping your body straight

Troubleshooting Tip: Adjust the angle of your body to make it more or less challenging. A more upright position is easier.

4. Doorway Chest Stretch (Upper Body) - 45 seconds

Steps:
1. Stand in an open doorway
2. Raise your arms to the sides at shoulder height
3. Place your palms on the door frame
4. Lean forward slightly until you feel a stretch in your chest
5. Hold this position, pressing your hands into the door frame

Troubleshooting Tip: If you can't reach the top of the doorway, lower your arms to a comfortable height.

5. Wall Sit (Lower Body) - 45 seconds

Steps:
1. Lean your back against a wall
2. Slide down until your thighs are parallel to the ground
3. Ensure your knees are above your ankles
4. Hold this position, keeping your core engaged

Troubleshooting Tip: If a full wall sit is too challenging, don't slide down as far. Even a slight bend in the knees will be beneficial.

6. Seated Spinal Twist (Core/Back) - 45 seconds

Steps:
1. Sit sideways in a chair with your feet flat on the floor
2. Twist your torso to face the back of the chair
3. Hold the back of the chair gently for support
4. Hold this twist, breathing deeply
5. Switch sides after 20 seconds

Troubleshooting Tip: Only twist as far as is comfortable. The goal is a gentle stretch and engagement, not maximum rotation.

7. Calf Raise Hold (Lower Body) - 45 seconds

Steps:
1. Stand behind a chair, holding it lightly for balance
2. Rise up onto your toes
3. Hold this position, keeping your core engaged
4. Focus on balance and stability

Troubleshooting Tip: If you can't rise fully onto your toes, even a small lift will engage your calf muscles.

8. Isometric Bicep Curl (Upper Body) - 45 seconds

Steps:
1. Sit in a chair with armrests
2. Place your hands under the armrests, palms facing up
3. Try to curl your arms upward, resisting with the armrests
4. Hold this contraction, feeling the engagement in your biceps

Troubleshooting Tip: If your chair doesn't have armrests, press your palms together in front of your chest instead.

9. Bird Dog Hold (Core/Back) - 45 seconds

Steps:
1. Start on your hands and knees on the floor (use a mat or towel for comfort)
2. Extend your right arm forward and left leg back
3. Hold this position, keeping your back flat and core engaged
4. Switch sides after 20 seconds

Troubleshooting Tip: If balance is challenging, keep both knees on the ground and just extend one arm at a time.

10. Isometric Shoulder Press (Upper Body) - 45 seconds

Steps:
1. Stand with your back against a wall
2. Raise your arms to shoulder height, bent at 90-degree angles
3. Press your arms back into the wall
4. Hold this position, engaging your shoulder and arm muscles

Troubleshooting Tip: If raising your arms to shoulder height is uncomfortable, perform the exercise at a lower height.

11. Standing Side Leg Lift (Lower Body) - 45 seconds

Steps:
1. Stand behind a chair, holding it for support
2. Lift your right leg out to the side
3. Hold for 5 seconds, then lower
4. Repeat with the left leg
5. Continue alternating sides

Troubleshooting Tip: Even a small lift will engage your hip muscles. Focus on control rather than height.

12. Stomach Vacuum (Core) - 45 seconds

Steps:
1. Stand or sit tall with good posture
2. Exhale fully, drawing your belly button towards your spine
3. Hold this "vacuum" position for as long as you can while taking small breaths
4. Relax and repeat

Troubleshooting Tip: If you feel lightheaded, take slightly deeper breaths or reduce the hold time.

Cool Down (2 minutes):
1. Gentle march in place for 30 seconds
2. Shoulder rolls: 5 backward, 5 forward
3. Gentle side-to-side neck tilts: 5 on each side
4. Deep breathing: Take 5 deep breaths, inhaling through your nose and exhaling through your mouth

Remember to drink water after completing your routine. This 20-minute strength builder is designed to challenge all major muscle groups through isometric contractions. As you become more comfortable with the routine, you can increase the difficulty by:

- Holding positions for longer durations
- Increasing the intensity of the contractions
- Adding small weights or resistance bands to some exercises (under guidance from a fitness professional)

Consistency is key – aim to perform this routine 2-3 times a week, allowing at least one day of rest between sessions. You'll likely notice improvements in your overall strength, endurance, and ability to perform daily activities with greater ease.

Always listen to your body and stop if you experience any pain or excessive discomfort. If you have any health concerns or medical conditions, consult with your healthcare provider before starting this or any new exercise routine.

Are you ready to build strength with this comprehensive isometric routine? Let's embark on this journey to a stronger, more capable you!

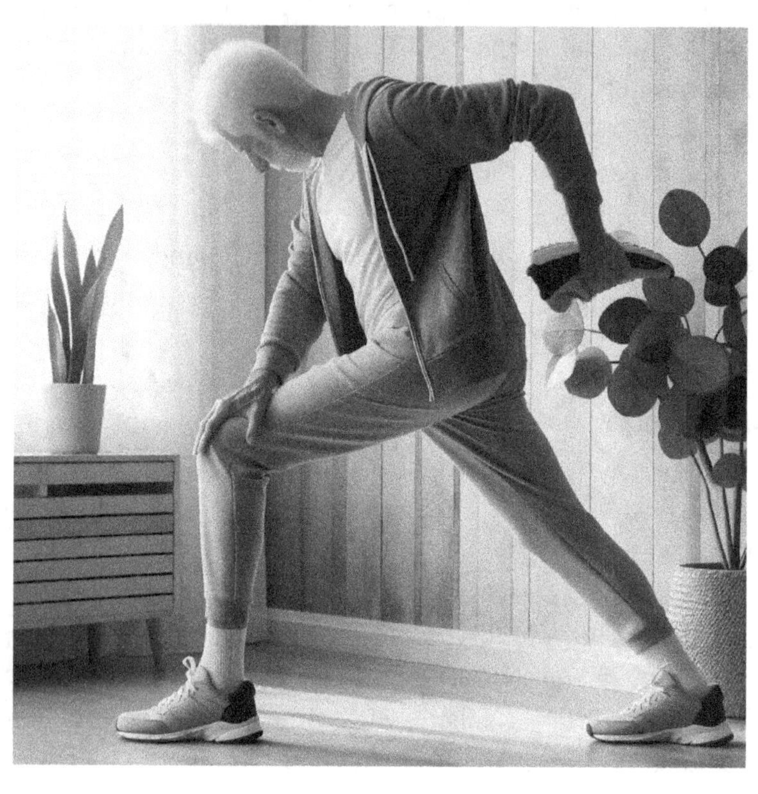

Arthritis and joint pain

Imagine finding relief from the stiffness and discomfort of arthritis, regaining some of the mobility and strength you may have lost. These exercises are designed to do just that, offering a way to stay active and manage pain without exacerbating your symptoms.

Before starting:
- Consult with your doctor or physical therapist to ensure these exercises are appropriate for your specific condition.
- Have a chair nearby for support.
- Keep a glass of water handy.
- Perform these exercises when your pain is at its lowest, typically later in the day.

Warm-Up (3 minutes):
1. Gentle marching in place for 30 seconds
2. Shoulder rolls: 5 forward, 5 backward
3. Gentle neck rotations: 5 in each direction
4. Ankle rotations: 5 circles in each direction with each foot
5. Wrist rotations: 5 circles in each direction with each hand

Now, let's move into the exercises. Perform each exercise for 10-15 seconds, gradually increasing to 30 seconds as you build strength. Rest for 15-30 seconds between exercises.

1. Hand Squeeze for Finger Arthritis

Steps:
1. Sit comfortably in a chair
2. Hold a soft stress ball or rolled-up sock in your hand
3. Gently squeeze the ball
4. Hold the squeeze for 5-10 seconds
5. Slowly release
6. Repeat 3-5 times with each hand

Troubleshooting Tip: If squeezing is too painful, try just holding the ball and focusing on keeping your grip steady.

2. Wrist Press for Wrist Arthritis

Steps:
1. Sit with your forearm resting on a table, palm down
2. Place your other hand on top of the resting hand
3. Gently press down with the top hand while resisting with the bottom hand
4. Hold for 5-10 seconds
5. Relax and repeat 3-5 times
6. Switch hands and repeat

Troubleshooting Tip: If this causes discomfort, reduce the pressure or try the exercise with your palm facing up instead.

3. Isometric Elbow Flexion for Elbow Arthritis

Steps:

1. Sit with your elbow bent at a 90-degree angle, palm facing up
2. Place your other hand on your wrist
3. Try to bend your elbow while resisting with your other hand
4. Hold for 5-10 seconds
5. Relax and repeat 3-5 times on each arm

Troubleshooting Tip: Adjust the angle of your elbow if 90 degrees is uncomfortable.

4. Isometric Shoulder External Rotation for Shoulder Arthritis

Steps:

1. Stand with your affected arm at your side, elbow bent to 90 degrees
2. Press the side of your fist against a wall
3. Try to rotate your arm outward while the wall provides resistance
4. Hold for 5-10 seconds
5. Relax and repeat 3-5 times on each side

Troubleshooting Tip: If standing is difficult, perform this seated with your elbow against the armrest of a chair.

5. Isometric Knee Extension for Knee Arthritis

Steps:
1. Sit in a chair with your back straight
2. Extend one leg out in front of you, foot slightly off the ground
3. Tighten your thigh muscles, trying to straighten your knee further
4. Hold for 5-10 seconds
5. Slowly lower your foot and relax
6. Repeat 3-5 times on each leg

Troubleshooting Tip: If extending your leg causes pain, keep your foot on the ground and focus on tightening your thigh muscle.

6. Ankle Press for Ankle Arthritis

Steps:
1. Sit in a chair with your feet flat on the floor
2. Press your toes into the ground while keeping your heel down
3. Hold for 5-10 seconds
4. Relax and repeat 3-5 times with each foot

Troubleshooting Tip: If this is too intense, try pressing with less force or alternating between pressing with your toes and your heel.

7. Hip Abduction for Hip Arthritis

Steps:
1. Stand holding onto a chair for balance
2. Lift your leg out to the side about 6 inches
3. Hold for 5-10 seconds
4. Slowly lower your leg
5. Repeat 3-5 times on each side

Troubleshooting Tip: If lifting your leg is too challenging, try pressing your leg outward against a wall instead.

8. Isometric Neck Flexion for Neck Arthritis

Steps:
1. Sit or stand with good posture
2. Place your hand on your forehead
3. Gently press your head forward into your hand while resisting with your hand
4. Hold for 5-10 seconds
5. Relax and repeat 3-5 times

Troubleshooting Tip: Use very gentle pressure to avoid strain. If this causes discomfort, skip this exercise and consult your doctor.

Cool Down (2 minutes):
1. Gentle shoulder shrugs: 5 repetitions
2. Deep breathing: Take 5 deep breaths, inhaling through your nose and exhaling through your mouth
3. Gentle finger and wrist stretches

Remember:

- Start with shorter hold times (5 seconds) and fewer repetitions, gradually increasing as you build strength and comfort.
- Perform these exercises 3-5 times per week, but listen to your body and rest when needed.
- Apply heat to your joints before exercising to increase flexibility, and ice afterward if you experience any swelling.
- If you experience increased pain that lasts for more than two hours after exercising, reduce the intensity or frequency of your routine.

These isometric exercises can help manage arthritis symptoms by strengthening the muscles around your joints, improving stability, and maintaining range of motion. However, it's crucial to work within your pain-free range and to stop if you experience any sharp or severe pain.

Remember, consistency is key. Even on days when your arthritis symptoms are more pronounced, try to do at least one or two of these exercises. Over time, you may notice improved joint function, reduced pain, and increased ability to perform daily activities.

Are you ready to take control of your arthritis symptoms with these gentle yet effective isometric exercises? Let's work together towards improved joint health and reduced pain!

Imagine maintaining strong bones and reducing your risk of fractures, even as you age. These exercises are designed to help you do just that, offering a safe way to stimulate bone growth and improve overall bone health.

Before starting:
- Consult with your doctor or physical therapist to ensure these exercises are appropriate for your condition.
- Wear comfortable, non-slip shoes.
- Have a sturdy chair and wall nearby for support.
- Keep a glass of water handy.

Warm-Up (3 minutes):
1. Gentle marching in place for 30 seconds
2. Arm circles: 5 forward, 5 backward
3. Gentle torso twists: 5 to each side
4. Ankle rotations: 5 circles in each direction with each foot
5. Shoulder shrugs: 5 repetitions

Now, let's move into the exercises. Perform each exercise for 15-20 seconds, gradually increasing to 30 seconds as you build strength. Rest for 15-30 seconds between exercises.

1. Wall Push for Upper Body Strength

Steps:
1. Stand arm's length from a wall
2. Place your palms flat against the wall at shoulder height
3. Lean in slightly and push against the wall

4. Hold this position, engaging your chest and arm muscles
5. Hold for 15-20 seconds, then relax
6. Repeat 2-3 times

Troubleshooting Tip: If your wrists feel strained, make fists and push with your knuckles instead.

2. Chair Squat Hold for Lower Body Strength

Steps:
1. Stand in front of a sturdy chair
2. Slowly lower yourself as if about to sit, stopping just before you touch the chair
3. Hold this position, keeping your weight in your heels
4. Keep your chest up and core engaged
5. Hold for 15-20 seconds, then slowly stand up
6. Repeat 2-3 times

Troubleshooting Tip: If holding the squat is too challenging, rest lightly on the chair while maintaining the squat position.

3. Single Leg Stand for Balance and Hip Strength

Steps:
1. Stand behind a chair, holding it lightly for support
2. Slowly lift your right foot off the ground
3. Hold this position for 15-20 seconds, focusing on keeping your standing leg straight
4. Lower your foot and repeat with the left leg
5. Perform 2-3 times on each side

Troubleshooting Tip: If lifting your foot is too challenging, start by just shifting your weight onto one leg while keeping both feet on the ground.

4. Wall Plank for Core and Spine Strength

Steps:
1. Stand facing a wall, about arm's length away
2. Place your forearms against the wall, elbows under shoulders
3. Lean forward, keeping your body in a straight line from head to heels
4. Push your forearms into the wall and engage your core
5. Hold for 15-20 seconds, then relax
6. Repeat 2-3 times

Troubleshooting Tip: Adjust the angle of your body to make it more or less challenging. A more upright position is easier.

5. Heel Raises for Ankle and Calf Strength

Steps:
1. Stand behind a chair, holding it lightly for balance
2. Slowly rise up onto your toes
3. Hold this position for 15-20 seconds
4. Slowly lower back down
5. Repeat 2-3 times

Troubleshooting Tip: If you can't rise fully onto your toes, even a small lift will be beneficial.

6. Isometric Chest Press for Upper Body Strength

Steps:
1. Stand in a doorway
2. Place your palms on either side of the doorframe at chest height
3. Push your hands into the doorframe as if trying to bring them together
4. Hold for 15-20 seconds, then relax
5. Repeat 2-3 times

Troubleshooting Tip: Adjust the height of your hands if shoulder level is uncomfortable.

7. Wall Sit for Leg and Core Strength

Steps:
1. Lean your back against a wall
2. Slide down until your thighs are parallel to the ground (or as low as comfortable)
3. Ensure your knees are above your ankles
4. Hold this position for 15-20 seconds
5. Slowly slide back up
6. Repeat 2-3 times

Troubleshooting Tip: If a full wall sit is too challenging, don't slide down as far. Even a slight bend in the knees will be beneficial.

8. Standing Row for Upper Back Strength

Steps:
1. Stand with your back against a wall
2. Bend your elbows and press the backs of your hands into the wall
3. Try to squeeze your shoulder blades together
4. Hold for 15-20 seconds, then relax
5. Repeat 2-3 times

Troubleshooting Tip: If reaching behind you is difficult, try this exercise seated in a chair, pressing your elbows back against the chair back.

Cool Down (2 minutes):
1. Gentle marching in place for 30 seconds
2. Deep breathing: Take 5 deep breaths, inhaling through your nose and exhaling through your mouth
3. Gentle stretches for calves, hamstrings, and chest

Remember:
- Perform these exercises 2-3 times per week, allowing at least one day of rest between sessions.
- Focus on maintaining good posture throughout all exercises.
- Increase the hold times gradually as you build strength and confidence.
- Always move slowly and controlled to prevent any sudden movements that could lead to injury.
- Stay hydrated and ensure you're getting adequate calcium and vitamin D in your diet to support bone health.

These isometric exercises can help improve bone density by creating tension in the muscles that pull on the bones. They also improve balance and strength, which are crucial for preventing falls - a major concern for those with osteoporosis.

It's important to note that while these exercises are generally safe for those with osteoporosis, everyone's condition is different. Always work within your pain-free range and stop if you experience any pain or discomfort.

Consistency is key when it comes to bone health. Even on days when you don't feel like exercising, try to do at least one or two of these exercises. Over time, you may notice improved strength, better balance, and increased confidence in your daily activities.

Are you ready to strengthen your bones and improve your overall health with these safe and effective isometric exercises? Let's work together towards better bone health and a more active lifestyle!

Imagine moving through your daily activities with confidence, free from the fear of falling. These exercises are designed to help you achieve just that, offering a safe way to improve your balance and reduce your risk of falls.

Before starting:
- Ensure you have a sturdy chair and wall nearby for support.
- Wear comfortable, non-slip shoes.
- Clear the area of any tripping hazards.
- Keep a glass of water handy.

Warm-Up (3 minutes):
1. Gentle marching in place for 30 seconds
2. Shoulder rolls: 5 forward, 5 backward
3. Ankle rotations: 5 circles in each direction with each foot
4. Gentle hip rotations: 5 in each direction
5. Head turns: Slowly look left, then right, 5 times each way

Now, let's move into the exercises. Perform each exercise for 15-20 seconds, gradually increasing to 30 seconds as you build strength and confidence. Rest for 15-30 seconds between exercises.

1. Single Leg Stand

Steps:
1. Stand behind a sturdy chair, holding it lightly for support
2. Slowly lift your right foot off the ground
3. Hold this position for 15-20 seconds, focusing on keeping your standing leg straight
4. Lower your foot and repeat with the left leg
5. Perform 2-3 times on each side

Troubleshooting Tip: If lifting your foot is too challenging, start by just shifting your weight onto one leg while keeping both feet on the ground.

2. Heel-to-Toe Walk

Steps:
1. Stand near a wall for support if needed
2. Place the heel of your right foot directly in front of the toes of your left foot
3. Take 5-10 steps forward in this manner, placing one foot directly in front of the other
4. Turn around carefully and return to the starting point

Troubleshooting Tip: If this is too difficult, start by just practicing the heel-to-toe stance without walking.

3. Clock Reach

Steps:
1. Imagine you're standing in the center of a clock face
2. Hold onto a chair with your left hand
3. Lift your right foot slightly off the ground
4. Extend your right arm to reach towards the numbers on the imaginary clock (12 o'clock, 3 o'clock, etc.)
5. Return to the center after each "number"
6. Repeat on the other side

Troubleshooting Tip: If balance is challenging, keep both feet on the ground and just practice reaching.

4. Wall Slide for Leg Strength

Steps:
1. Stand with your back against a wall
2. Slowly slide down the wall until your thighs are parallel to the ground (or as low as comfortable)
3. Hold this position for 15-20 seconds
4. Slowly slide back up
5. Repeat 2-3 times

Troubleshooting Tip: If a full slide is too challenging, only go down a short distance. Even a slight bend in the knees will be beneficial.

5. Toe and Heel Raises

Steps:

1. Stand behind a chair, holding it lightly for support
2. Rise up onto your toes and hold for 5 seconds
3. Lower back down
4. Rock back onto your heels, lifting your toes off the ground, and hold for 5 seconds
5. Return to the starting position
6. Repeat this sequence 3-5 times

Troubleshooting Tip: If you can't lift your heels or toes very high, even a small movement will help improve ankle strength and flexibility.

6. Standing Core Engagement

Steps:

1. Stand with your feet hip-width apart
2. Place your hands on your hips
3. Imagine pulling your belly button towards your spine
4. Hold this engagement for 15-20 seconds while breathing normally
5. Relax and repeat 2-3 times

Troubleshooting Tip: If you're unsure about engaging your core, imagine preparing for someone to gently punch your stomach.

7. Flamingo Stand

Steps:
1. Stand on your right leg, holding a chair for support
2. Bend your left knee, bringing your foot behind you
3. Hold this position for 15-20 seconds, focusing on keeping your standing leg straight
4. Lower your foot and repeat on the other side
5. Perform 2-3 times on each side

Troubleshooting Tip: If you can't lift your foot behind you, simply shift your weight onto one leg while keeping both feet on the ground.

8. Chair Sit-to-Stand

Steps:
1. Sit in a chair with your feet flat on the floor
2. Slowly stand up, using your hands on the armrests if needed
3. Once standing, hold the position for 5 seconds
4. Slowly sit back down
5. Repeat 5-8 times

Troubleshooting Tip: If standing fully is challenging, practice just lifting your bottom off the chair slightly and holding that position.

Cool Down (2 minutes):

1. Gentle marching in place for 30 seconds
2. Shoulder rolls: 5 backward, 5 forward
3. Ankle rotations: 5 circles in each direction with each foot
4. Deep breathing: Take 5 deep breaths, inhaling through your nose and exhaling through your mouth

Remember:

- Perform these exercises 3-4 times per week.
- Always have a stable support nearby when practicing balance exercises.
- Increase the duration and difficulty of the exercises gradually as you build confidence.
- Focus on maintaining good posture throughout all exercises.
- If you feel dizzy or unsteady at any point, stop the exercise and rest.

These exercises are designed to improve your balance by strengthening the muscles that keep you stable, enhancing your proprioception, and improving your overall body awareness. Regular practice can significantly reduce your risk of falls.

It's important to be patient with yourself. Balance improves gradually with consistent practice. Even if you can only do these exercises for a short time at first, you're making progress!

In addition to these exercises, consider these fall prevention tips:

- Keep your home well-lit and free of clutter
- Use non-slip mats in the bathroom and kitchen
- Wear properly fitting, supportive shoes
- Have your vision and hearing checked regularly
- Review your medications with your doctor, as some can affect balance

Are you ready to improve your balance and reduce your risk of falls with these safe and effective exercises? Let's work together towards a steadier, more confident you!

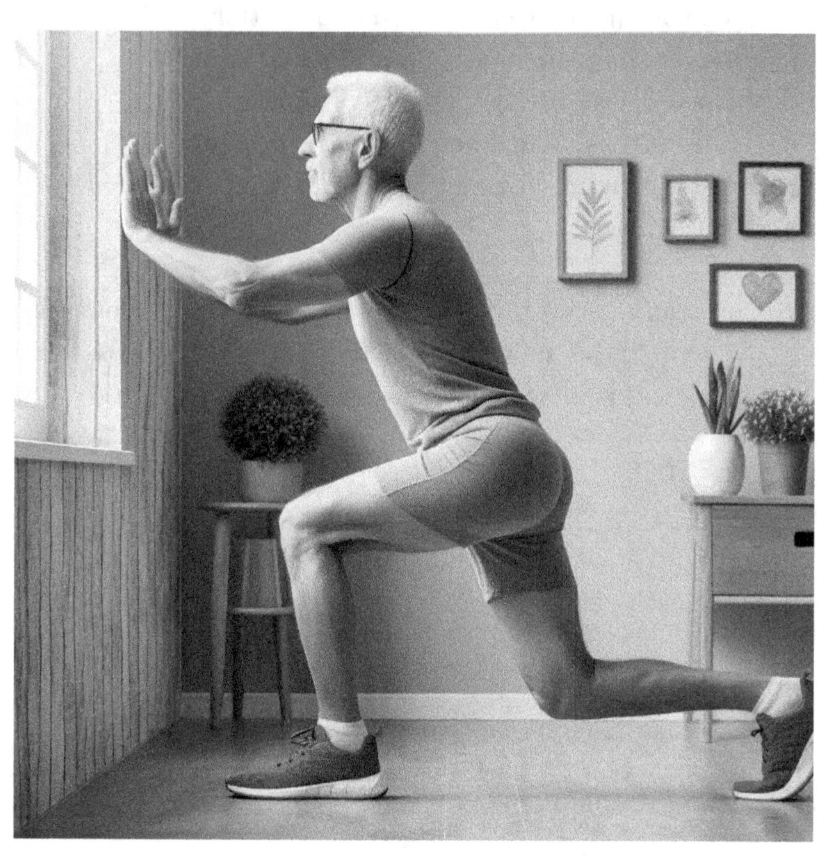

Imagine being able to maintain your strength and flexibility even during long periods of sitting, whether at your desk or on a long journey. These exercises are designed to help you do just that, offering a way to stay active and healthy even in sedentary situations.

Before starting:
- Ensure you're seated comfortably with your feet flat on the floor.
- Maintain good posture throughout the exercises.
- Breathe normally during each exercise.
- If you're in an office chair with wheels, make sure it's stable and won't roll.

1. Isometric Abdominal Contraction

Steps:
1. Sit up straight in your chair.
2. Take a deep breath in.
3. As you exhale, tighten your abdominal muscles, pulling your navel towards your spine.
4. Hold this contraction for 5-10 seconds while breathing normally.
5. Relax and repeat 5-8 times.

Troubleshooting Tip: If you're not sure you're engaging your abs correctly, place your hand on your stomach to feel the muscles tighten.

2. Seated Glute Squeeze

Steps:
1. Sit up straight in your chair.
2. Squeeze your buttocks together as tightly as you can.
3. Hold this contraction for 5-10 seconds.
4. Relax and repeat 8-10 times.

Troubleshooting Tip: If you have trouble feeling this, try shifting your weight slightly forward in the chair.

3. Neck Press

Steps:
1. Place your right hand on the right side of your head.
2. Gently press your head into your hand while resisting with your hand.
3. Hold for 5-10 seconds.
4. Repeat on the left side.
5. Do 3-5 repetitions on each side.

Troubleshooting Tip: Use very gentle pressure to avoid strain. If this causes any discomfort, skip this exercise.

4. Shoulder Blade Squeeze

Steps:
1. Sit up straight with your arms relaxed at your sides.
2. Slowly squeeze your shoulder blades together.
3. Hold this position for 5-10 seconds.
4. Slowly relax.
5. Repeat 5-8 times.

Troubleshooting Tip: Imagine trying to hold a pencil between your shoulder blades to get the right movement.

5. Hand and Forearm Strengthener

Steps:
1. Hold your hands out in front of you, palms facing each other.
2. Press your palms together firmly.
3. Hold this pressure for 10-15 seconds.
4. Relax and repeat 5-8 times.

Troubleshooting Tip: If this causes wrist discomfort, try pressing your fingertips together instead.

6. Seated Leg Extension

Steps:
1. Sit up straight with your feet flat on the floor.
2. Slowly lift your right foot until your leg is as straight as comfortable.
3. Hold this position for 5-10 seconds, focusing on tightening your thigh muscle.

4. Slowly lower your foot back to the ground.
5. Repeat with your left leg.
6. Do 5-8 repetitions with each leg.

Troubleshooting Tip: If you can't fully extend your leg, lift it as high as comfortable. The key is to feel the contraction in your thigh.

7. Ankle Rotations and Holds

Steps:
1. Lift your right foot slightly off the ground.
2. Rotate your ankle in a circular motion 5 times clockwise, then 5 times counterclockwise.
3. Point your toes forward and hold for 5 seconds.
4. Flex your foot (toes towards shin) and hold for 5 seconds.
5. Repeat with your left foot.

Troubleshooting Tip: If you experience any cramping, gently massage your calf and take a short break before continuing.

8. Seated Spinal Twist

Steps:
1. Sit sideways in your chair.
2. Twist your torso to face the back of the chair.
3. Place your hands on the back of the chair for support.
4. Hold this twist for 10-15 seconds, breathing deeply.
5. Slowly return to the starting position and repeat on the other side.

Troubleshooting Tip: Only twist as far as is comfortable. The goal is a gentle stretch, not maximum rotation.

9. Isometric Bicep Curl

Steps:
1. If your chair has armrests, place your hands under them, palms facing up.
2. Push up against the armrests as if trying to do a bicep curl.
3. Hold this contraction for 10-15 seconds.
4. Relax and repeat 3-5 times.

Troubleshooting Tip: If your chair doesn't have armrests, you can press your palms together in front of your chest instead.

10. Seated Knee Press

Steps:
1. Sit up straight with your feet flat on the floor.
2. Press your knees together as firmly as you can.
3. Hold this contraction for 10-15 seconds.
4. Relax and repeat 5-8 times.

Troubleshooting Tip: Place a small pillow or rolled-up jacket between your knees to increase resistance.

Remember:

- You can perform these exercises individually throughout the day or as a complete routine.
- Aim to do this routine 2-3 times during a long day of sitting.
- Listen to your body and stop if you experience any pain or discomfort.
- Stay hydrated, especially when traveling.
- Take breaks to stand up and walk around when possible, even if it's just for a minute or two.

These seated isometric exercises can help maintain muscle tone, improve circulation, and reduce stiffness associated with prolonged sitting. They're especially beneficial during long flights, car rides, or office days when movement is limited.

By incorporating these exercises into your daily routine, you're taking an important step in maintaining your health and mobility, even in situations where traditional exercise isn't possible.

Are you ready to turn your seat into a subtle workout space? Let's make the most of those sedentary moments and keep your body active and healthy!

Imagine turning your everyday household tasks into opportunities for improving your strength and balance. These exercises are designed to seamlessly integrate with your chores, allowing you to multitask for your health.

Before starting:
- Wear comfortable, non-slip shoes.
- Ensure your environment is clear of tripping hazards.
- Listen to your body and stop if you feel any pain or excessive discomfort.

1. Counter Push-Ups While Waiting for Water to Boil

Steps:
1. Stand arm's length from your kitchen counter.
2. Place your hands shoulder-width apart on the edge of the counter.
3. Lean in, bending your elbows slightly.
4. Push against the counter for 10-15 seconds.
5. Relax and repeat 3-5 times.

Troubleshooting Tip: Adjust your body angle to make it easier or more challenging. A more upright position is easier.

2. Calf Raises While Washing Dishes

Steps:
1. Stand at the sink with feet hip-width apart.
2. Slowly rise up onto your toes.

3. Hold this position for 10-15 seconds.
4. Slowly lower back down.
5. Repeat 5-8 times.

Troubleshooting Tip: If balance is an issue, keep one hand on the counter for support.

3. Wall Sit While Folding Laundry

Steps:
1. Lean your back against a wall near your laundry area.
2. Slide down until your thighs are parallel to the ground (or as low as comfortable).
3. Hold this position while folding a few items of clothing.
4. Slide back up and rest for a moment.
5. Repeat 2-3 times during your laundry session.

Troubleshooting Tip: If a full wall sit is too challenging, don't slide down as far. Even a slight bend in the knees is beneficial.

4. Single Leg Stand While Brushing Teeth

Steps:
1. Stand near your bathroom sink for support if needed.
2. Shift your weight onto your right leg.
3. Lift your left foot slightly off the ground.
4. Hold this position while brushing your teeth.
5. Switch legs halfway through brushing.

Troubleshooting Tip: If lifting your foot is too challenging, just shift your weight onto one leg while keeping both feet on the ground.

5. Doorway Chest Stretch While Waiting for Laundry/Dishwasher

Steps:
1. Stand in an open doorway.
2. Raise your arms to the sides at shoulder height.
3. Place your palms on the door frame.
4. Lean forward slightly until you feel a stretch in your chest.
5. Hold this position for 15-30 seconds.
6. Repeat 2-3 times.

Troubleshooting Tip: If you can't reach the top of the doorway, lower your arms to a comfortable height.

6. Core Engagement While Vacuuming or Sweeping

Steps:
1. As you vacuum or sweep, stand tall with good posture.
2. Engage your core by pulling your navel towards your spine.
3. Hold this engagement as you move around cleaning.
4. Focus on maintaining the contraction for 30-60 seconds at a time.
5. Relax and repeat throughout your cleaning session.

Troubleshooting Tip: If you're unsure about engaging your core, imagine preparing for someone to gently punch your stomach.

7. Glute Squeezes While Walking Up Stairs

Steps:

1. As you climb stairs, focus on squeezing your buttocks with each step.
2. Hold the squeeze for a moment at the top of each step.
3. Continue this throughout your climb.

Troubleshooting Tip: If you don't have stairs, you can do this while stepping up onto a curb or low step.

8. Isometric Shoulder Press While Reaching for High Shelves

Steps:

1. When reaching for a high shelf, press your hands up against the shelf.
2. Hold this press for 5-10 seconds.
3. Slowly release and retrieve the item you need.
4. Repeat whenever reaching for high items.

Troubleshooting Tip: Only reach for items at a comfortable height. Never strain or overreach, especially for heavy objects.

9. Wall Push While Waiting for Microwave

Steps:
1. Stand arm's length from a wall near your microwave.
2. Place your palms flat against the wall at shoulder height.
3. Lean in slightly and push against the wall.
4. Hold this push for the duration of the microwave timer.
5. Relax when the microwave beeps.

Troubleshooting Tip: If your wrists feel strained, make fists and push with your knuckles instead.

10. Toe Taps While Watching TV Commercials

Steps:
1. Stand behind your couch or a sturdy chair for support.
2. Lift your right foot and tap your toe out to the side.
3. Return to center and repeat with your left foot.
4. Continue alternating for the duration of a commercial break.

Troubleshooting Tip: If balance is challenging, keep both feet on the ground and just shift your weight side to side.

Remember:
- Integrate these exercises naturally into your routine. Don't force them if you're in a hurry or the situation isn't safe.
- Focus on maintaining good posture throughout your chores.

- These exercises can be done individually or combined, depending on your tasks and energy level.
- Stay hydrated, especially when doing more active chores.
- Take breaks if you feel fatigued.

By incorporating these isometric exercises into your chores, you're maximizing your time and taking care of both your home and your health. It's a great way to stay active, especially on days when you might not have time for a dedicated workout.

Are you ready to turn your household tasks into opportunities for strength and balance training? Let's make your chores work double-duty for your health!

Imagine ending your day with a series of calming exercises that release tension, quiet your mind, and prepare your body for deep, restorative sleep. This routine is designed to do just that, combining gentle isometric contractions with relaxation techniques.

Before starting:
- Perform this routine in your bedroom or a quiet, comfortable space.
- Wear loose, comfortable clothing.
- Have a pillow nearby for support if needed.
- Dim the lights to create a relaxing atmosphere.

1. Seated Deep Breathing (2 minutes)

Steps:
1. Sit comfortably on the edge of your bed.
2. Close your eyes and place one hand on your chest, the other on your belly.
3. Inhale slowly through your nose for a count of 4, feeling your belly expand.
4. Hold your breath for a count of 4.
5. Exhale slowly through your mouth for a count of 6.
6. Repeat this cycle for 2 minutes.

Troubleshooting Tip: If you feel lightheaded, return to your normal breathing pattern and try again with shorter counts.

2. Neck and Shoulder Release (1 minute each side)

Steps:
1. Remain seated and drop your right ear towards your right shoulder.
2. Place your right hand gently on the left side of your head.
3. Apply very gentle pressure with your hand while slightly resisting with your neck.
4. Hold for 5 seconds, then relax for 5 seconds.
5. Repeat 3 times, then switch to the left side.

Troubleshooting Tip: If you experience any neck pain, skip this exercise and consult with your healthcare provider.

3. Seated Spinal Twist (30 seconds each side)

Steps:
1. Sit sideways on your bed with your feet flat on the floor.
2. Twist your torso to the right, placing your left hand on your right knee.
3. Place your right hand behind you for support.
4. Hold this gentle twist for 30 seconds, breathing deeply.
5. Slowly return to center and repeat on the left side.

Troubleshooting Tip: Only twist as far as is comfortable. The goal is gentle stretching, not maximum rotation.

4. Lying Leg Press (1 minute)

Steps:
1. Lie on your back on your bed with your knees bent, feet flat.

2. Lift your right foot off the bed and press it against your left hand.

3. Apply gentle pressure with your hand while pushing with your foot.

4. Hold for 5 seconds, then relax for 5 seconds.

5. Repeat 3 times, then switch legs.

Troubleshooting Tip: If lifting your leg is uncomfortable, try this exercise with both feet on the bed, pressing your feet into the mattress.

5. Abdominal Breathing with Engagement (2 minutes)

Steps:

1. Lie on your back with your knees bent, feet flat on the bed.

2. Place your hands on your lower abdomen.

3. As you inhale, let your belly expand into your hands.

4. As you exhale, gently draw your navel towards your spine.

5. Hold this gentle contraction for 2-3 seconds, then relax.

6. Continue this pattern for 2 minutes.

Troubleshooting Tip: If you feel any strain in your lower back, place a pillow under your knees.

6. Progressive Muscle Relaxation (5 minutes)

Steps:
1. Lie comfortably on your back.
2. Starting with your toes, tense the muscles for 5 seconds, then relax for 10 seconds.
3. Move up to your calves, thighs, buttocks, abs, hands, arms, shoulders, neck, and face.
4. Tense and relax each muscle group in turn.
5. Finish by taking three deep breaths.

Troubleshooting Tip: If tensing any muscle group causes pain, simply focus on relaxing that area without the initial tension.

7. Mindful Body Scan (3 minutes)

Steps:
1. Remain lying on your back with your eyes closed.
2. Bring your attention to your toes and gradually move up your body.
3. Notice any sensations or areas of tension without trying to change them.
4. Spend about 10-15 seconds on each body part.
5. End by taking three deep breaths, imagining relaxation spreading throughout your body.

Troubleshooting Tip: If your mind wanders, gently bring your focus back to the body part you were scanning.

8. Gratitude Reflection (1 minute)

Steps:
1. Still lying down, bring to mind three things you're grateful for from your day.
2. They can be big or small – a tasty meal, a kind word, a beautiful sunset.
3. Spend a few moments really feeling the gratitude in your body.

Troubleshooting Tip: If you're having trouble thinking of things, start with basic blessings like having a bed to sleep in or the ability to breathe.

Cool Down:
Take three final deep breaths, exhaling fully each time. Allow yourself to settle into a comfortable position for sleep.

Remember:
- Perform this routine consistently, ideally every night.
- If you don't have time for the full routine, even doing a few of these exercises can be beneficial.
- Focus on the sensation of relaxation spreading through your body.
- If you find yourself getting sleepy before finishing the routine, that's okay – let yourself drift off to sleep.

This bedtime relaxation routine combines gentle isometric exercises with relaxation techniques to help release physical tension and calm your mind. By practicing regularly, you may find that you fall asleep more easily and enjoy more restful sleep.

Are you ready to transform your bedtime routine into a relaxing, rejuvenating experience? Let's prepare your body and mind for a night of restorative sleep!

Imagine steadily building your strength and endurance, allowing you to perform daily activities with greater ease and confidence. This progression plan is designed to help you safely and effectively advance your isometric training.

Before starting:
- Ensure you've been consistently performing isometric exercises for at least 4-6 weeks.
- Always warm up before exercising and cool down afterward.
- Listen to your body and progress at a pace that feels challenging but manageable.

Step-by-Step Guide to Progression:

1. Establish Your Baseline

Steps:
1. Choose 3-5 key isometric exercises you perform regularly.
2. Note your current hold time and perceived effort for each exercise.
3. Use a scale of 1-10 to rate your effort, where 1 is very easy and 10 is maximum effort.

Example:
- Wall sit: 20 seconds, effort level 6/10
- Plank: 15 seconds, effort level 7/10
- Doorway chest press: 10 seconds, effort level 5/10

Troubleshooting Tip: If you're unsure about rating your effort, focus on how challenging the exercise feels in the last few seconds of your hold.

2. Increase Duration

Steps:
1. Start by increasing your hold time by 2-5 seconds for each exercise.
2. Maintain this new duration for 1-2 weeks before increasing again.
3. Aim to increase duration by 10-20% every 1-2 weeks.

Example:
Week 1-2: Wall sit for 22-25 seconds
Week 3-4: Wall sit for 24-27 seconds

Troubleshooting Tip: If you can't maintain proper form for the increased duration, it's okay to drop back to your previous hold time and progress more slowly.

3. Increase Intensity

Steps:
1. Once you can hold an exercise for 30-45 seconds with good form, focus on increasing intensity rather than duration.

2. To increase intensity, apply more force during the isometric hold.

3. Your hold time may decrease initially as you increase intensity - this is normal.

Example:

For a wall push:

- Push more forcefully against the wall
- Rate your effort level and aim to increase it by 1-2 points

Troubleshooting Tip: Increase intensity gradually. If you feel any pain or excessive strain, reduce the force and build up more slowly.

4. Add Sets

Steps:

1. Start by adding one additional set of each exercise.
2. Rest for 30-60 seconds between sets.
3. Gradually increase to 3-5 sets of each exercise.

Example:

Week 1: 2 sets of 20-second wall sits

Week 3: 3 sets of 20-second wall sits

Troubleshooting Tip: If you feel fatigued before completing all sets, it's okay to reduce the duration or intensity for the later sets.

5. Incorporate Unilateral Exercises

Steps:
1. Once comfortable with bilateral exercises, try unilateral (one-sided) versions.
2. Start with a shorter duration than your bilateral exercises.
3. Ensure you perform equal repetitions on both sides.

Example:
Progress from a two-legged wall sit to a single-leg wall sit, starting with half the duration.

Troubleshooting Tip: Use support (like a chair or wall) when first attempting unilateral exercises to ensure safety.

6. Use Progressive Overload

Steps:
1. Gradually increase one variable (duration, intensity, or sets) every 1-2 weeks.
2. Focus on progressing 1-2 exercises at a time rather than all exercises simultaneously.
3. Track your progress in a journal or app.

Example:
Week 1-2: Increase wall sit duration
Week 3-4: Increase plank intensity
Week 5-6: Add a set to doorway chest press

Troubleshooting Tip: If you hit a plateau, try varying your routine or taking a deload week where you reduce intensity before progressing again.

7. Incorporate Timed Challenges

Steps:
1. Once a month, test how long you can hold key exercises.
2. Record your times and try to beat them in future challenges.
3. Ensure you maintain proper form throughout the challenge.

Example:
Monthly challenge: How long can you hold a wall sit?

Troubleshooting Tip: Stop the challenge if your form begins to deteriorate or if you feel any pain.

8. Listen to Your Body

Steps:
1. Pay attention to how your body feels during and after exercises.
2. If you experience pain or excessive fatigue, scale back your progression.
3. Allow for adequate rest between training sessions (usually 24-48 hours).

Troubleshooting Tip: If you're consistently feeling overly fatigued, consider reducing the frequency of your workouts or the rate of progression.

Remember:
- Progress should be gradual and consistent.
- It's normal to have some weeks where you don't see improvement - this is part of the process.
- Celebrate small victories along the way.
- Stay hydrated and maintain a balanced diet to support your training.
- Consider consulting with a physical therapist or certified fitness professional for personalized progression strategies.

By following this progression plan, you'll continue to challenge your muscles and make steady gains in strength and endurance. This approach helps prevent plateaus and keeps your workouts engaging and effective.

Are you ready to take your isometric training to the next level? Let's steadily build your strength and endurance for improved daily function and overall health!

Imagine enhancing your strength routine with movements that more closely mimic daily activities. This approach will help you build functional strength and improve your overall mobility.

Before starting:
- Ensure you have a solid foundation in basic isometric exercises.
- Wear comfortable, supportive shoes.
- Have a chair or wall nearby for support if needed.
- Always warm up before exercising and cool down afterward.

Step-by-Step Guide to Adding Dynamic Movements:

1. Isometric Hold to Dynamic Movement

Exercise: Wall Sit to Squat

Steps:
1. Start with a standard wall sit, holding for 10-15 seconds.
2. Slowly push through your heels to stand up.
3. Lower back down into the wall sit position.
4. Repeat 5-8 times.

Troubleshooting Tip: If full squats are challenging, start by only coming up halfway before lowering back down.

2. Alternating Isometric Holds

Exercise: Alternating Leg Raises

Steps:
1. Sit in a chair with good posture.
2. Lift your right leg and hold for 5 seconds.
3. Lower your right leg and immediately lift your left leg.
4. Hold for 5 seconds.
5. Continue alternating for 8-10 repetitions per leg.

Troubleshooting Tip: If lifting your leg is difficult, start by just sliding your foot forward on the ground.

3. Isometric Hold with Small Movement

Exercise: Plank with Arm Lift

Steps:
1. Start in a forearm plank position (on knees if needed).
2. Hold the plank for 10 seconds.
3. Slowly lift your right arm off the ground.
4. Hold for 2-3 seconds, then lower.
5. Repeat with the left arm.
6. Continue alternating for 5-6 lifts per arm.

Troubleshooting Tip: If arm lifts are too challenging, start by just shifting your weight slightly to one side at a time.

4. Isometric to Dynamic and Back

Exercise: Wall Push to Arm Circles

Steps:
1. Start with a wall push, holding for 10 seconds.
2. Step back from the wall and do 5 small arm circles forward.
3. Return to the wall push for another 10 seconds.
4. Step back and do 5 small arm circles backward.
5. Repeat this sequence 3-4 times.

Troubleshooting Tip: Keep the arm circles small at first, gradually increasing the size as you get comfortable with the movement.

5. Adding Movement to Balance Exercises

Exercise: Single Leg Stand with Leg Swings

Steps:
1. Stand on your right leg, holding onto a chair for support if needed.
2. Hold this position for 10 seconds.
3. Slowly swing your left leg forward and back 5 times.
4. Return to the static single leg stand for another 10 seconds.
5. Repeat on the other side.

Troubleshooting Tip: Start with very small leg swings, focusing on maintaining balance throughout the movement.

6. Isometric Pulses

Exercise: Chair Dips with Pulses

Steps:
1. Sit on the edge of a sturdy chair with your hands gripping the edge on either side of your hips.
2. Slide your buttocks off the chair, supporting your weight with your arms.
3. Hold this position for 5 seconds.
4. Do 5 small pulses, lowering and raising your body about an inch.
5. Return to the static hold for another 5 seconds.
6. Repeat 3-4 times.

Troubleshooting Tip: Keep your feet closer to the chair to make the exercise easier, or further away to make it more challenging.

7. Dynamic Movement to Isometric Hold

Exercise: Marching to Knee Hold

Steps:
1. Stand tall with good posture.
2. March in place for 10 steps, lifting your knees high.
3. On the last step, hold your knee up for 10 seconds.
4. Lower and repeat, holding the other knee up for 10 seconds.
5. Repeat this sequence 3-4 times.

Troubleshooting Tip: If holding your knee up is challenging, use a wall or chair for support.

8. Adding Resistance to Isometric Holds

Exercise: Wall Sit with Water Bottle Press

Steps:
1. Hold a water bottle in each hand.
2. Perform a wall sit and hold for 10 seconds.
3. While maintaining the wall sit, press the water bottles out to the sides.
4. Hold this position for 5 seconds.
5. Bring the water bottles back in and hold the wall sit for another 10 seconds.
6. Repeat 3-4 times.

Troubleshooting Tip: Start with partially filled water bottles and gradually increase the water level as you get stronger.

Remember:
- Introduce these dynamic movements gradually, one or two at a time.
- Focus on maintaining good form throughout both the isometric holds and dynamic movements.
- Progress slowly, mastering each movement before moving on to more challenging variations.
- Listen to your body and stop if you experience any pain or excessive discomfort.
- Stay hydrated and take breaks as needed.

- Aim to incorporate these combination exercises 2-3 times per week, allowing for rest days in between.

By adding these dynamic movements to your isometric routine, you'll improve your functional strength, enhance your balance and coordination, and add variety to your workouts. This approach helps bridge the gap between static strength and the movements required in daily life.

Are you ready to add some dynamic flair to your isometric training? Let's get moving and take your strength and mobility to the next level!

Imagine having a diverse fitness routine that improves your strength, flexibility, cardiovascular health, and overall well-being. By combining isometric exercises with other forms of exercise, you can achieve a comprehensive workout regimen tailored to your needs and preferences.

Before starting:
- Consult with your healthcare provider before significantly changing your exercise routine.
- Ensure you have a good foundation in basic isometric exercises.
- Have appropriate equipment for the additional exercise forms you'll be incorporating.
- Listen to your body and progress at a comfortable pace.

Step-by-Step Guide to Combining Exercise Forms:

1. Isometrics with Cardiovascular Exercise

Combination: Walking with Isometric Intervals

Steps:
1. Start with a 5-minute warm-up walk at a comfortable pace.
2. Walk at a moderate pace for 2 minutes.
3. Stop and perform a wall sit for 15-30 seconds.
4. Resume walking for another 2 minutes.
5. Stop and do a standing calf raise hold for 15-30 seconds.
6. Continue alternating 2 minutes of walking with different isometric holds.

7. Cool down with a 5-minute easy walk.

Troubleshooting Tip: If you're just starting, use shorter walking intervals and isometric hold times, gradually increasing as you build stamina.

2. Isometrics with Yoga

Combination: Sun Salutation with Isometric Plank

Steps:
1. Perform a standard sun salutation sequence.
2. When you reach the plank position, hold it isometrically for 10-15 seconds.
3. Continue with the rest of the sun salutation.
4. Repeat the sequence 3-5 times, incorporating different isometric holds (like chair pose or warrior pose) in each round.

Troubleshooting Tip: If holding poses is challenging, use props like blocks or a chair for support.

3. Isometrics with Resistance Band Training

Combination: Resistance Band Row with Isometric Hold

Steps:
1. Secure a resistance band to a sturdy object at chest height.
2. Grasp the band handles and step back until there's tension in the band.

3. Perform a rowing motion, pulling the handles towards your chest.

4. At the end of the row, hold the position isometrically for 5-10 seconds.

5. Slowly return to the starting position.

6. Repeat 8-12 times.

Troubleshooting Tip: Start with a lighter resistance band and shorter isometric holds, progressing as you build strength.

4. Isometrics with Balance Training

Combination: Single Leg Stand with Arm Movements

Steps:

1. Stand on your right leg, lifting your left foot slightly off the ground.

2. Hold this balance for 10 seconds.

3. While maintaining balance, slowly raise your arms out to the sides.

4. Hold this position isometrically for 5-10 seconds.

5. Lower your arms and then your foot.

6. Repeat on the other side.

7. Perform 3-5 repetitions per leg.

Troubleshooting Tip: Stand near a wall or chair for support if needed, gradually reducing your reliance on support as your balance improves.

5. Isometrics with Pilates

Combination: Pilates Hundred with Isometric Leg Lift

Steps:
1. Lie on your back with your legs in tabletop position (knees bent, shins parallel to the floor).
2. Lift your head, neck, and shoulders off the mat.
3. Extend your arms by your sides, palms facing down.
4. Pump your arms up and down in small movements for a count of 50.
5. At count 50, straighten your legs and lift them about 45 degrees off the mat.
6. Hold this position isometrically for 10-15 seconds while continuing to pump your arms.
7. Lower your legs and upper body to rest.

Troubleshooting Tip: If holding your legs up is too challenging, keep them in the tabletop position or lower them closer to the ground.

6. Isometrics with Stretching

Combination: Hamstring Stretch with Isometric Contraction

Steps:
1. Sit on the floor with your right leg extended and your left leg bent, foot against your right inner thigh.
2. Reach towards your right foot, feeling a stretch in your hamstring.
3. Hold the stretch for 15 seconds.

4. Now, try to press your heel into the floor while maintaining the stretch position.
5. Hold this isometric contraction for 5-10 seconds.
6. Relax and deepen the stretch for another 15 seconds.
7. Repeat on the other side.

Troubleshooting Tip: If you can't reach your foot, use a towel or strap around your foot to help you maintain the stretch position.

7. Isometrics with Functional Training

Combination: Farmer's Walk with Isometric Pauses

Steps:
1. Hold a weight (like a water bottle or dumbbell) in each hand by your sides.
2. Walk forward for 10 steps.
3. Stop and hold your position, engaging your core and arm muscles isometrically for 10 seconds.
4. Resume walking for another 10 steps.
5. Stop and perform a calf raise hold for 10 seconds.
6. Continue this pattern for 3-5 minutes.

Troubleshooting Tip: Start with light weights and short distances, gradually increasing as you build strength and endurance.

Remember:

- Introduce new exercise combinations gradually, allowing your body to adapt.
- Maintain proper form in both the isometric and dynamic portions of each exercise.
- Stay hydrated and listen to your body, taking rest days as needed.
- Aim for a balanced routine that includes strength, flexibility, and cardiovascular elements.
- Modify exercises as necessary to suit your fitness level and any physical limitations.

By combining isometric exercises with other forms of exercise, you're creating a well-rounded fitness routine that addresses multiple aspects of physical health. This approach can help improve overall strength, flexibility, balance, and cardiovascular fitness while keeping your workouts varied and engaging.

Are you excited to diversify your workout routine? Let's blend isometrics with other exercise forms for a comprehensive approach to your fitness journey!

Protein needs for muscle maintenance

Imagine maintaining strong, healthy muscles well into your golden years, supporting your active lifestyle and independence. Proper protein intake is crucial for this goal, especially for seniors engaging in regular exercise.

Step-by-Step Guide to Meeting Protein Needs:

1. Understand Your Protein Requirements

Steps:
1. Calculate your body weight in kilograms (divide your weight in pounds by 2.2).
2. Multiply your weight in kg by 1.2-1.5 grams of protein.
3. This gives you your daily protein need in grams.

Example: A 150-pound senior would need about 82-102 grams of protein daily.

Troubleshooting Tip: If you have kidney issues, consult your doctor before increasing protein intake.

2. Distribute Protein Intake Throughout the Day

Steps:
1. Divide your daily protein need by 3-4 meals.
2. Aim to consume this amount of protein at each meal.
3. Include a protein source with snacks as well.

Example: For 90 grams daily, aim for about 25-30 grams per meal.

Troubleshooting Tip: If large meals are difficult, have smaller, more frequent protein-rich meals or snacks.

3. Choose High-Quality Protein Sources

Steps:
1. Include lean meats like chicken, turkey, or fish in your meals.
2. Incorporate eggs, either whole or egg whites.
3. Use dairy products like Greek yogurt or cottage cheese.
4. Include plant-based proteins like beans, lentils, and tofu.

Troubleshooting Tip: If chewing meat is difficult, try ground meats, fish, or plant-based alternatives.

4. Optimize Protein Timing

Steps:
1. Consume a protein-rich meal or snack within 30 minutes after exercise.
2. Include protein in your bedtime snack to support overnight muscle recovery.

Example: Have a small serving of Greek yogurt with berries before bed.

Troubleshooting Tip: If you're not hungry after exercise, try a protein shake or smoothie.

5. Use Protein Supplements When Necessary

Steps:
1. Choose a high-quality protein powder (whey, casein, or plant-based).
2. Mix 1 scoop (typically 20-25 grams of protein) with water or milk.
3. Use as a snack or to boost protein content of meals.

Troubleshooting Tip: If you experience digestive issues with protein powders, try different types or consult a dietitian.

6. Incorporate Protein-Rich Snacks

Steps:
1. Keep hard-boiled eggs in the fridge for a quick snack.
2. Prepare small containers of nuts and seeds for on-the-go protein.
3. Stock up on Greek yogurt or cottage cheese for easy, protein-rich options.

Troubleshooting Tip: If nuts are hard to chew, try nut butters spread on whole grain crackers or fruit.

7. Balance Protein with Other Nutrients

Steps:

1. Include a variety of colorful fruits and vegetables in your diet.
2. Choose whole grains for added fiber and nutrients.
3. Include healthy fats like avocado, olive oil, and fatty fish.

Troubleshooting Tip: If you have trouble eating a variety of foods, consider a high-quality multivitamin (consult your doctor first).

8. Stay Hydrated

Steps:

1. Drink water with every meal and snack.
2. Aim for at least 8 cups (64 ounces) of fluid daily.
3. Increase intake during and after exercise.

Troubleshooting Tip: If plain water is unappealing, try infusing it with fruit or herbs for flavor.

9. Monitor Your Progress

Steps:

1. Keep a food diary for a week to track your protein intake.
2. Note how you feel in terms of energy and muscle soreness.
3. Adjust your intake based on your observations and energy levels.

Troubleshooting Tip: Use a smartphone app to easily track your protein intake if keeping a written diary is cumbersome.

10. Consult Professionals When Needed

Steps:
1. Discuss your protein needs with your doctor, especially if you have any health conditions.
2. Consider working with a registered dietitian for personalized nutrition advice.
3. Consult a certified fitness professional to ensure your exercise routine supports your nutrition goals.

Troubleshooting Tip: If professional consultations are costly, look for community health programs or senior centers that may offer nutrition guidance.

Remember:
- Gradual changes are often more sustainable than drastic ones.
- Listen to your body and adjust your intake as needed.
- Protein needs may increase with more intense exercise or if you're recovering from illness or injury.
- Quality of protein is just as important as quantity.
- Stay consistent with both your nutrition and exercise routine for best results.

By following these steps, you can ensure you're meeting your protein needs to support muscle maintenance and overall health as a senior athlete. Proper protein intake, combined with regular exercise, can help you maintain strength, support recovery, and enhance your overall quality of life.

Are you ready to fuel your active lifestyle with optimal protein intake? Let's nourish those muscles and support your athletic endeavors well into your golden years!

Imagine maintaining optimal performance, preventing fatigue, and supporting your overall health through proper hydration and electrolyte balance. This is especially important for seniors, as the body's ability to regulate fluid balance can change with age.

Step-by-Step Guide to Maintaining Hydration and Electrolyte Balance:

1. Understand Your Hydration Needs

Steps:
1. Calculate your base water need: divide your weight in pounds by 2, this gives you the ounces of water to drink daily.
2. Add 12 ounces for every 30 minutes of exercise.

Example: A 150-pound senior needs about 75 ounces of water daily, plus extra for exercise.

Troubleshooting Tip: If you have heart or kidney issues, consult your doctor for personalized hydration recommendations.

2. Create a Hydration Schedule

Steps:
1. Start your day with a glass of water.
2. Drink a glass of water with each meal.

3. Have a water bottle nearby and sip regularly throughout the day.
4. Drink before, during, and after exercise.

Troubleshooting Tip: If you often forget to drink, set reminders on your phone or use a marked water bottle to track intake.

3. Recognize Signs of Dehydration

Steps:
1. Check your urine color - aim for pale yellow.
2. Be aware of symptoms like dry mouth, fatigue, or dizziness.
3. Monitor your weight before and after exercise - significant drops indicate fluid loss.

Troubleshooting Tip: If you're unsure about your hydration status, consult your doctor or a sports nutritionist.

4. Incorporate Hydrating Foods

Steps:
1. Eat water-rich fruits like watermelon, oranges, and grapes.
2. Include hydrating vegetables such as cucumbers, tomatoes, and lettuce in your meals.
3. Have soups or broths, especially in cooler weather.

Troubleshooting Tip: If chewing fruits is difficult, try making smoothies or eating softer fruits like berries.

5. Balance Electrolytes

Steps:
1. Include sodium: add a pinch of salt to your water during intense exercise.
2. Consume potassium-rich foods like bananas, sweet potatoes, and yogurt.
3. Get magnesium from nuts, seeds, and leafy greens.
4. Ensure calcium intake through dairy or fortified plant-based alternatives.

Troubleshooting Tip: If you're on a low-sodium diet, consult your doctor about electrolyte balance during exercise.

6. Use Sports Drinks Wisely

Steps:
1. For exercise lasting less than an hour, water is usually sufficient.
2. For longer or more intense sessions, consider a sports drink.
3. Choose low-sugar options or dilute regular sports drinks with water.

Troubleshooting Tip: If commercial sports drinks cause digestive issues, try making your own with water, a pinch of salt, and a splash of juice.

7. Adjust for Weather Conditions

Steps:

1. Increase fluid intake in hot or humid weather.
2. Don't forget to hydrate in cold weather, even if you don't feel as thirsty.
3. Be extra vigilant about hydration at high altitudes.

Troubleshooting Tip: In extreme conditions, weigh yourself before and after exercise to gauge fluid loss and replace accordingly.

8. Pre-hydrate Before Exercise

Steps:

1. Drink 16-20 ounces of water 2-3 hours before exercise.
2. Have another 8 ounces 20-30 minutes before starting.
3. Ensure you're well-hydrated but not uncomfortable.

Troubleshooting Tip: If pre-exercise hydration causes discomfort, try smaller sips over a longer period.

9. Hydrate During Exercise

Steps:

1. Aim for 7-10 ounces of fluid every 10-20 minutes during exercise.
2. For longer sessions, alternate between water and an electrolyte drink.
3. Adjust intake based on exercise intensity and weather conditions.

Troubleshooting Tip: If drinking during exercise is challenging, practice taking small sips during your workouts.

10. Rehydrate Post-Exercise

Steps:
1. Weigh yourself before and after exercise.
2. For every pound lost, drink 16-24 ounces of fluid.
3. Include a small amount of salt and carbohydrates to aid absorption.

Troubleshooting Tip: If you struggle to drink enough after exercise, try hydrating foods like fruit or soup.

11. Monitor Medications and Hydration

Steps:
1. Be aware that some medications can affect hydration needs.
2. Consult your doctor about how your medications might impact fluid balance.
3. Adjust your hydration strategy accordingly.

Troubleshooting Tip: Keep a list of your medications and their potential effects on hydration to share with your healthcare providers.

Remember:
- Thirst is not always a reliable indicator of hydration needs, especially for seniors.

- Consistent, regular hydration is more effective than trying to catch up all at once.
- Over-hydration is possible, so balance is key.
- Hydration needs can vary based on individual factors, activity level, and climate.
- Regular weigh-ins can help you track your hydration status.

By following these steps, you can maintain proper hydration and electrolyte balance, supporting your performance as a senior athlete and promoting overall health. Proper hydration is crucial for temperature regulation, joint lubrication, nutrient transport, and overall bodily functions.

Are you ready to optimize your hydration strategy and maintain electrolyte balance? Let's keep your body well-hydrated and performing at its best, no matter your age or activity level!

Imagine maintaining your fitness routine while giving your body the time it needs to repair, rebuild, and grow stronger. Proper rest and active recovery are crucial components of any successful training program, especially for senior athletes.

Step-by-Step Guide to Rest and Active Recovery:

1. Understand the Importance of Rest

Steps:
1. Recognize that rest is when your body repairs and strengthens itself.
2. Accept that rest days are as important as workout days.
3. Learn to listen to your body's signals for needed rest.

Troubleshooting Tip: If you feel guilty about taking rest days, remind yourself that they're essential for progress and injury prevention.

2. Implement a Sleep Routine

Steps:
1. Aim for 7-9 hours of sleep per night.
2. Establish a consistent bedtime and wake-up time.
3. Create a relaxing pre-sleep routine (e.g., reading, gentle stretching).
4. Keep your bedroom cool, dark, and quiet.

Troubleshooting Tip: If you have trouble falling asleep, try a white noise machine or app to create a soothing environment.

3. Practice Active Recovery

Steps:
1. On rest days, engage in light, low-impact activities.
2. Try a gentle walk for 20-30 minutes.
3. Perform easy stretching or yoga poses.
4. Go for a leisurely swim or water aerobics session.

Troubleshooting Tip: If you're tempted to push too hard during active recovery, set a "perceived effort" limit of 3-4 out of 10.

4. Incorporate Flexibility Work

Steps:
1. Dedicate time to stretching major muscle groups daily.
2. Hold each stretch for 15-30 seconds.
3. Focus on areas that feel tight or sore.
4. Consider trying a gentle yoga class designed for seniors.

Troubleshooting Tip: If traditional stretching is uncomfortable, try dynamic stretches or foam rolling instead.

5. Use Proper Cool-Down Techniques

Steps:
1. After each workout, spend 5-10 minutes cooling down.
2. Gradually reduce the intensity of your activity.

3. Perform light stretches for the muscles you've worked.

4. Take deep, calming breaths to help your body transition to rest.

Troubleshooting Tip: If you're short on time, at least walk slowly for a few minutes post-workout rather than stopping abruptly.

6. Practice Stress-Reduction Techniques

Steps:

1. Learn and practice deep breathing exercises.

2. Try progressive muscle relaxation.

3. Consider meditation or mindfulness practices.

4. Engage in hobbies or activities you find relaxing.

Troubleshooting Tip: If traditional meditation is challenging, try a guided relaxation app or video.

7. Use Cold and Heat Therapy

Steps:

1. Apply ice to sore muscles for 15-20 minutes after intense workouts.

2. Use heat therapy before exercise to loosen tight muscles.

3. Consider alternating between cold and heat for chronic issues.

4. Always wrap ice or heat packs in a towel to protect your skin.

Troubleshooting Tip: If you're unsure about using cold or heat, consult with a physical therapist for personalized advice.

8. Implement Regular Massage or Self-Massage

Steps:
1. Schedule regular massage sessions if possible.
2. Learn self-massage techniques for major muscle groups.
3. Use foam rollers or massage balls for self-myofascial release.
4. Start gently and gradually increase pressure as tolerated.

Troubleshooting Tip: If traditional massage is too intense, try gentler techniques like effleurage or lymphatic drainage.

9. Monitor and Manage Fatigue

Steps:
1. Keep a log of your energy levels and workout performance.
2. Note any persistent fatigue or decrease in performance.
3. Adjust your training schedule if you notice ongoing fatigue.
4. Consider reducing workout intensity or frequency if needed.

Troubleshooting Tip: If fatigue persists despite adequate rest, consult your healthcare provider to rule out underlying issues.

10. Plan Recovery Weeks

Steps:
1. Every 4-6 weeks, schedule a recovery week.
2. Reduce your workout volume and intensity by about 40-50%.
3. Focus on technique and form rather than pushing hard.
4. Use this time to assess your progress and set new goals.

Troubleshooting Tip: If a full recovery week feels too long, try a 3-4 day "mini-recovery" period instead.

11. Stay Socially Active

Steps:
1. Engage in light social activities on rest days.
2. Join a seniors' walking group or gentle exercise class.
3. Spend time with friends and family.
4. Pursue hobbies that are mentally stimulating but physically relaxing.

Troubleshooting Tip: If in-person social activities are challenging, consider virtual options like online clubs or video calls with friends.

Remember:
- Recovery needs can vary greatly between individuals.
- Listen to your body and adjust your recovery strategies as needed.
- Consistency in recovery is as important as consistency in training.

- Over-resting can lead to deconditioning, so balance is key.
- If you're unsure about your recovery needs, consult with a fitness professional experienced in working with seniors.

By implementing these rest and active recovery strategies, you can support your body's repair processes, prevent burnout, and maintain your fitness journey as a senior athlete. Proper recovery allows you to come back to your workouts feeling refreshed and ready to make progress.

Are you ready to prioritize recovery and give your body the care it needs? Let's make rest and active recovery integral parts of your fitness routine, ensuring you can stay active and healthy for years to come!

Keeping an exercise journal

Imagine having a clear record of your fitness journey, allowing you to see your progress, identify patterns, and stay motivated over time. An exercise journal can be a powerful tool for achieving your fitness goals and maintaining enthusiasm for your workouts.

Step-by-Step Guide to Keeping an Exercise Journal:

1. Choose Your Journal Format

Steps:
1. Decide between a physical notebook or a digital app.
2. For a physical journal, choose one that's portable and has enough space for daily entries.
3. If going digital, consider apps like MyFitnessPal, Fitbit, or a simple notes app on your smartphone.

Troubleshooting Tip: If you're not tech-savvy, start with a physical journal. You can always transition to a digital format later.

2. Set Up Your Journal Structure

Steps:
1. Create sections for different types of information (e.g., daily workouts, weekly summaries, goals).
2. Include space for date, time, and type of exercise.
3. Add columns for duration, intensity, and how you felt during/after the workout.
4. Leave room for additional notes or observations.

Troubleshooting Tip: If structuring your journal feels overwhelming, start simple with just date, exercise, and duration. You can add more details as you get comfortable.

3. Record Your Baseline Measurements

Steps:
1. Note your starting weight, if relevant to your goals.
2. Measure and record key body measurements (e.g., waist, hips, chest).
3. Perform and record results from baseline fitness tests (e.g., how long you can hold a wall sit, number of chair stands in 30 seconds).
4. Write down your current energy levels and any physical limitations.

Troubleshooting Tip: If you're uncomfortable with body measurements, focus on functional fitness tests or simply how you feel day-to-day.

4. Set Clear, Achievable Goals

Steps:
1. Write down your short-term (1-3 months) and long-term (6-12 months) fitness goals.
2. Make sure your goals are SMART (Specific, Measurable, Achievable, Relevant, Time-bound).
3. Break larger goals into smaller, manageable milestones.

Troubleshooting Tip: If you're unsure about setting appropriate goals, consult with a fitness professional or your healthcare provider.

5. Log Your Daily Workouts

Steps:
1. Immediately after each workout, record the date and type of exercise.
2. Note the duration and intensity of your workout.
3. Write down any specific exercises performed, including repetitions and sets if applicable.
4. Record how you felt during and after the workout.

Troubleshooting Tip: If you forget to log immediately, set a daily reminder on your phone to fill in your journal.

6. Track Your Progress

Steps:
1. Weekly: Review your journal entries and summarize your week's activities.

2. Monthly: Retake your baseline measurements and fitness tests.

3. Note any improvements or changes in your abilities or how you feel.

4. Adjust your goals if necessary based on your progress.

Troubleshooting Tip: If you're not seeing the progress you expected, don't get discouraged. Use this information to reassess and adjust your approach.

7. Monitor Your Recovery

Steps:

1. Note your sleep quality and duration each night.

2. Record any muscle soreness or fatigue.

3. Track your energy levels throughout the day.

4. Note how well you're recovering between workouts.

Troubleshooting Tip: If you consistently feel overly fatigued, it might be a sign to incorporate more rest or decrease workout intensity.

8. Include Nutrition Information

Steps:

1. Write down what you eat before and after workouts.

2. Note how different foods affect your energy and performance.

3. Track your water intake, especially on workout days.

Troubleshooting Tip: If detailed food tracking feels overwhelming, start by just noting pre and post-workout meals.

9. Record Non-Exercise Activities

Steps:
1. Note any physical activities outside of planned workouts (e.g., gardening, house chores).
2. Record your daily step count if you use a pedometer or fitness tracker.
3. Include any recreational activities or sports you participate in.

Troubleshooting Tip: If you don't have a step counter, estimate your activity level (low, moderate, high) for the day.

10. Reflect and Adjust

Steps:
1. At the end of each week, write a brief reflection on your progress and challenges.
2. Note what's working well and what might need adjustment.
3. Set focus areas or goals for the coming week.
4. Celebrate your successes, no matter how small.

Troubleshooting Tip: If you're struggling to stay consistent, try setting a specific time each week for reflection and planning.

Remember:

- Be honest in your journal entries – it's for your benefit.
- Consistency is key – try to write in your journal daily, even if it's just a brief note.
- Your journal is personal – include whatever information is most helpful and motivating for you.
- Use your journal as a tool for accountability and motivation.
- Look back at your earlier entries periodically to see how far you've come.

By keeping an exercise journal, you create a powerful tool for tracking your fitness journey, identifying patterns, and staying motivated. It can help you celebrate your progress, adjust your approach when needed, and maintain your commitment to a healthy, active lifestyle.

Are you ready to start documenting your fitness journey? Let's begin your exercise journal today and watch your progress unfold over time!

Measuring improvements in strength and flexibility

Imagine being able to quantify your progress, seeing concrete evidence of how your hard work is paying off. Measuring improvements in strength and flexibility can provide motivation and help you adjust your training program as needed.

Step-by-Step Guide to Measuring Strength and Flexibility:

1. Establish Baseline Measurements

Steps:
1. Choose a day when you're well-rested and not sore from recent workouts.
2. Perform each test in the same order each time you measure.
3. Record your initial measurements in your exercise journal.
4. Date your entries for future reference.

Troubleshooting Tip: If you're unsure about proper form for any test, consult a fitness professional or physical therapist.

2. Strength Test: Chair Stand Test

Steps:
1. Sit in a sturdy chair with your feet flat on the floor.
2. Cross your arms over your chest.
3. Stand up and sit down as many times as you can in 30 seconds.

4. Count and record the number of full stands.

Troubleshooting Tip: If you can't stand without using your arms, note this and count how many stands you can do with arm assistance.

3. Strength Test: Wall Push-Up Test

Steps:
1. Stand arm's length from a wall.
2. Place your hands flat against the wall at shoulder height.
3. Perform as many wall push-ups as you can with good form.
4. Count and record the number completed.

Troubleshooting Tip: If wall push-ups are too easy, try them on a sturdy counter or the back of a couch for more challenge.

4. Flexibility Test: Sit and Reach

Steps:
1. Sit on the floor with your legs straight out in front of you.
2. Place a yardstick between your legs, with the 15-inch mark at your heels.
3. Reach forward as far as you can, sliding your hands along the yardstick.
4. Record the farthest point you can reach and hold for 2 seconds.

Troubleshooting Tip: If sitting on the floor is uncomfortable, try this test while sitting on the edge of a chair, reaching towards your toes.

5. Flexibility Test: Back Scratch Test

Steps:
1. Stand up straight.
2. Reach one arm over your shoulder and down your back.
3. Reach the other arm behind your back and up, trying to touch your fingers.
4. Measure the distance between your fingertips (overlap is positive, gap is negative).
5. Repeat on the other side.

Troubleshooting Tip: Use a ruler or ask someone to help you measure if you can't see the distance yourself.

6. Balance Test: Single Leg Stand

Steps:
1. Stand near a wall or chair for safety.
2. Lift one foot off the ground, bending your knee.
3. Time how long you can hold this position (up to 60 seconds).
4. Record your time and repeat with the other leg.

Troubleshooting Tip: If 60 seconds is too easy, try closing your eyes during the test for an added challenge.

7. Cardiovascular Endurance: 2-Minute Step Test

Steps:
1. Mark a point on the wall at the level of your hip bone.
2. March in place for 2 minutes, lifting your knees to the marked point.
3. Count how many times your right foot touches the ground.
4. Record your total count.

Troubleshooting Tip: If you need to stop before 2 minutes, record the time you stopped and your count at that point.

8. Grip Strength Test (if you have access to a hand dynamometer)

Steps:
1. Hold the dynamometer in your hand, arm at a 90-degree angle.
2. Squeeze as hard as you can for 5 seconds.
3. Record the measurement.
4. Repeat with the other hand.

Troubleshooting Tip: If you don't have a dynamometer, track how long you can hold a heavy book or filled water jug with each hand.

9. Schedule Regular Retests

Steps:
1. Set a schedule for retesting, typically every 4-6 weeks.
2. Perform the tests under similar conditions each time (time of day, warm-up, etc.).
3. Record new measurements in your exercise journal.
4. Compare to your baseline and previous measurements.

Troubleshooting Tip: If you're not seeing improvements, don't get discouraged. Use this information to reassess your training program.

10. Analyze Your Results

Steps:
1. Look for trends in your measurements over time.
2. Note which areas are showing the most improvement.
3. Identify areas that might need more focus in your training.
4. Celebrate your progress, no matter how small.

Troubleshooting Tip: If you're having trouble interpreting your results, consider sharing them with a fitness professional for insight.

11. Adjust Your Training Program

Steps:
1. Based on your results, identify areas needing more work.
2. Increase the challenge in exercises where you're seeing good progress.

3. Consider adding new exercises to target areas lagging in improvement.

4. Set new goals based on your progress.

Troubleshooting Tip: If you're unsure how to adjust your program, consult with a fitness professional experienced in working with seniors.

Remember:

- Consistency in how you perform the tests is crucial for accurate comparisons.
- Improvements may be gradual, especially as we age. Celebrate all progress.
- These tests measure different aspects of fitness. You may see more progress in some areas than others.
- Always prioritize safety. If a test feels unsafe, modify it or skip it.
- Use these measurements as motivation, not discouragement.

By regularly measuring your strength and flexibility, you can track your progress over time, adjust your fitness program as needed, and stay motivated by seeing concrete improvements. Remember, the goal is progress, not perfection.

Are you ready to start quantifying your fitness journey? Let's begin measuring your strength and flexibility to celebrate your progress and guide your future training!

Imagine continuously evolving your fitness journey, always having something new to strive for and achieve. Setting appropriate goals and challenges can keep your fitness routine exciting and motivating, helping you to maintain and improve your health and abilities over time.

Step-by-Step Guide to Setting New Goals and Challenges:

1. Reflect on Your Current Progress

Steps:
1. Review your exercise journal and recent fitness test results.
2. Note areas where you've made significant progress.
3. Identify areas that may need more attention.
4. Consider how your current fitness level aligns with your overall health goals.

Troubleshooting Tip: If you're having trouble assessing your progress objectively, consider discussing your results with a fitness professional or your healthcare provider.

2. Identify Your Motivations

Steps:
1. Ask yourself why fitness is important to you at this stage of life.
2. List specific benefits you hope to gain or maintain (e.g., independence, energy, specific activities you enjoy).

3. Consider any upcoming life events that might influence your fitness goals (e.g., travel plans, family events).

Troubleshooting Tip: If you're struggling to identify motivations, try visualizing your ideal day and how improved fitness could enhance it.

3. Set SMART Goals

Steps:
1. Specific: Clearly define what you want to achieve.
2. Measurable: Ensure you can quantify your progress.
3. Achievable: Make sure the goal is realistic given your current fitness level.
4. Relevant: Align the goal with your overall health and lifestyle objectives.
5. Time-bound: Set a specific timeframe for achieving the goal.

Example SMART Goal: "I will be able to perform 15 chair stands in 30 seconds by the end of three months, improving from my current 10 stands."

Troubleshooting Tip: If you're new to SMART goals, start with just one or two to avoid feeling overwhelmed.

4. Create a Mix of Short-term and Long-term Goals

Steps:
1. Set 1-2 short-term goals (achievable in 4-6 weeks).
2. Establish 1-2 medium-term goals (3-6 months).

3. Define 1 long-term goal (6 months to 1 year).
4. Ensure your short and medium-term goals support your long-term objective.

Troubleshooting Tip: If you're unsure about appropriate timelines, consult with a fitness professional who can help you set realistic expectations.

5. Include Various Fitness Components

Steps:
1. Set goals related to cardiovascular endurance (e.g., walking distance or duration).
2. Include strength-related goals (e.g., number of chair stands or wall push-ups).
3. Add flexibility goals (e.g., improving your sit-and-reach score).
4. Consider balance and coordination goals (e.g., increasing single-leg stand time).

Troubleshooting Tip: If you excel in one area but struggle in others, focus more goals on your weaker areas while maintaining your strengths.

6. Incorporate Lifestyle Goals

Steps:
1. Set goals related to consistency (e.g., exercising 3 times per week).
2. Include nutrition-related goals if relevant (e.g., increasing daily protein intake).

3. Consider sleep and recovery goals (e.g., establishing a consistent sleep schedule).

Troubleshooting Tip: Start with small, easily achievable lifestyle goals to build confidence and momentum.

7. Create Challenges to Keep Things Interesting

Steps:
1. Set up a personal challenge (e.g., try a new type of exercise each month).
2. Join or create a group challenge with friends or at your local senior center.
3. Consider signing up for an event like a charity walk to train towards.

Troubleshooting Tip: If group activities aren't possible, create virtual challenges with friends or family members.

8. Break Down Larger Goals into Milestones

Steps:
1. Identify key steps needed to reach your larger goals.
2. Create mini-goals or milestones for each step.
3. Set dates for achieving each milestone.

Example: If your goal is to walk a 5K, set milestones for distance increases every two weeks.

Troubleshooting Tip: If you miss a milestone, don't get discouraged. Adjust your timeline and keep moving forward.

9. Write Down Your Goals and Share Them

Steps:
1. Record your goals in your exercise journal.
2. Share your goals with a friend, family member, or fitness buddy.
3. Consider posting your goals somewhere visible as a daily reminder.

Troubleshooting Tip: If you're private about your goals, share with just one trusted person who can offer support and accountability.

10. Plan Your Approach

Steps:
1. Outline the specific actions needed to achieve each goal.
2. Identify any resources you might need (e.g., equipment, classes, information).
3. Schedule your workouts and activities in your calendar.

Troubleshooting Tip: If you're unsure about the best approach, consider consulting a fitness professional for guidance.

11. Regular Review and Adjustment

Steps:
1. Set a recurring date (e.g., monthly) to review your goals.
2. Assess your progress towards each goal.

3. Adjust goals as needed based on your progress and any changes in your health or circumstances.
4. Celebrate achievements and set new goals as you reach current ones.

Troubleshooting Tip: If you find yourself consistently missing goals, they might be too ambitious. It's okay to adjust them to be more achievable.

Remember:
- Goals should be challenging but attainable.
- It's okay to adjust your goals as you progress or if circumstances change.
- Celebrate all achievements, no matter how small.
- Use setbacks as learning opportunities, not reasons to give up.
- Your journey is unique – avoid comparing your goals or progress to others.

By setting new goals and challenges, you create a roadmap for your fitness journey that keeps you engaged, motivated, and continuously improving. Remember, the process of working towards your goals is just as important as achieving them.

Are you ready to set some exciting new fitness goals and challenges? Let's chart the course for the next phase of your fitness journey and watch as you continue to grow stronger and healthier!

www.ingramcontent.com/pod-product-compliance
Lightning Source LLC
Chambersburg PA
CBHW051558250726
48653CB00004BA/1209